For Darian

In the best of health,

Dr. Murray.

NATURAL BABY— HEALTHY CHILD

ALTERNATIVE HEALTH CARE SOLUTIONS FROM PRE-CONCEPTION THROUGH CHILDHOOD

FROM ALLERGIES TO AUTISM, ASTHMA, EAR INFECTIONS, COLDS, FLUS, AND ADD/ADHD

THE ULTIMATE GUIDE FOR NATURAL HEALING AND REMEDIES

DR. MURRAY CLARKE

D0961734

Natural Baby – Healthy Child: Alternative Health Care Solutions from Pre-conception Through Childhood – From Allergies to Autism, Asthma, Ear Infections, Colds, Flus, and ADD/ADHD – The Ultimate Guide for Natural Healing and Remedies

By Murray Clarke

1. Health & Fitness : Pregnancy & Childbirth 2. Family & Relationships : Health - General 3. Health & Fitness : Children's Health

ISBN: 978-1-935953-05-0

Cover design by Lewis Agrell

Printed in the United States of America

Authority Publishing

11230 Gold Express Dr. #310-413

Gold River, CA 95670

800-877-1097

www.AuthorityPublishing.com

Acknowledgements

This book is the result of many great teachers along the way, including and most importantly, the many families and parents who have entrusted the care of their children in my hands. Thank you.

In taking this book from my mind and into what you hold in front of you I would particularly like to thank Dora Lendvai, whose assistance in my clinic and with this book is invaluable and golden. I would like to thank Harvey Rosenfield for his fine mind and editorial suggestions which made this a better book. I feel extremely fortunate to have had Andrea Hurst guiding the course of this book with her masterful agent's balance of insight, experience and practicality, and for recommending Barry Fox who sculpted my original manuscript into a working text. Thank you also to Stephanie Chandler and Amberly Finarelli at Authority Publishing for their effortless expertise and finesse.

In the realm of healing and medicine I have had the good fortune to study with the homeopathic master Vega Rozenberg, whose wisdom and knowledge are also woven throughout this book.

Preface

This book is written to educate parents so they can be assisted in addressing the fact that today's children are the unhealthiest generation of children in modern times.

Despite being born into unprecedented affluence and supposedly advanced medical care, the last forty years has seen an epidemic rise in American children who suffer from chronic health conditions, increasing from 2 percent to 18 percent of the childhood population. This is an extraordinary 900 percent increase; it means that almost one in five American children will live with compromised health for the rest of their lives unless they seek and apply the attributes of holistic medicine.

This huge increase in the number of children afflicted with these chronic health problems is not confined to America. This is a global phenomenon and we now see the same increases in all these disorders affecting children in Europe, Asia, Australia and New Zealand.

Parents in America and around the world are aware that their children are suffering in ever-increasing numbers, and are actively looking for solutions and medical care that are alternatives to the standard pharmaceutical approach provided by traditional M.D. pediatricians.

At a very appropriate time, this book identifies and documents the underlying dietary, environmental, medical forces and factors that are contributing to this worldwide decline in children's health.

This is followed by a presentation of solutions that all parents can apply, with ease and confidence, to correct, enhance and protect their child's health, starting with pre-conception preparation by the mother, into pregnancy, the baby's first year and on throughout childhood.

The rich range of options is presented in a detailed but easily and quickly referenced style. These options include diet, environmental detoxification, nutritional supplementation, and holistic modalities including homeopathy, naturopathy, osteopathy, chiropractic and acupuncture. Parents will gain an intimate understanding of how to select and apply these methods for their child's benefit and good health.

I found a fruitful world, because my ancestors planted it for me. Likewise I am planting for my children.

—Talmud, Ta'anit 23a.

Table of Contents

Introduction

During the last forty plus years, American children have enjoyed unprecedented affluence, in addition to what is typically considered "advanced" medical care known as "allopathic" care. Yet at the same time, the number of children in the United States suffering from chronic health conditions— medical problems that will affect them for the rest of their lives—has increased *ninefold*, skyrocketing from 2 percent of the childhood population in 1960 to 18 percent today.[1] That's nearly one in five children!

In just the past 15 to 25 years, chronic conditions like ADD (Attention Deficit Disorder) and ADHD (Attention Deficit/Hyperactivity Disorder) have increased by 400 percent, autism by 300 percent[2], childhood allergies by 300 percent[3], asthma by 200 percent[4], and ear infections by 135 percent (with 69 percent of American children experiencing at least one such infection[5]). Today in America, one in three children is overweight or obese[6], and for the first time in history we are seeing children with high blood pressure and type 2 (adult-onset) diabetes at levels reaching epidemic proportions.[7] Unfortunately, the problem is not limited

to America: children throughout Europe, Asia, Australia and
New Zealand, are also suffering these same illnesses at the same
rates. Type 2 diabetes, for example, is expected to increase ten
times during the next decade among children living in the U.S.,
England and Europe[8] In one of the largest children's study of
its kind, "The worldwide time trends in asthma, allergies and
eczema in childhood" reported the same extreme increases for
these disorders in countries all around the world.[9] Forty years
ago, the first survey of autism in England indicated that 1 in 2,500
children suffered from this disorder.[10] Today, we now see that 1
in every 150 children in America, England, Europe and Japan are
autistic.[11,12] The number of children in Australia and New Zealand
with this severe disorder is just slightly less, with 1 in every 250
children diagnosed with autism.[13] Taken together, these alarming
facts make it abundantly clear that today's children are the sickest
generation in modern times.[14]

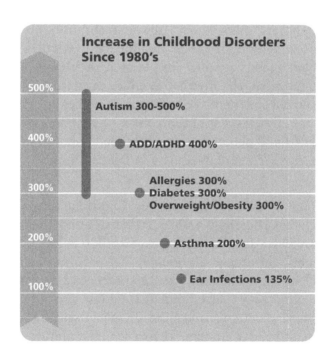

Increase in Childhood Disorders Since 1980's

500%

Autism 300-500%

400%

ADD/ADHD 400%

300%

Allergies 300%
Diabetes 300%
Overweight/Obesity 300%

200%

Asthma 200%

100%

Ear Infections 135%

When we see so many children from so many countries around the world suffering from these disorders, we see that there must be some common denominators and stresses that are affecting children so deeply and creating such alarming increases in these conditions.

There is no doubt that the underlying causes of these chronic diseases include our polluted environment, unnatural diet, sedentary lifestyle, misguided allopathic/pharmaceutical medical treatments and elevated stress levels. This generation of children has been exposed to more man-made environmental, dietary and pharmaceutical stressors than any since the beginning of human life. Lead, dioxins and hydrocarbons are found in every breath of air. Petrochemicals, pesticides and pharmaceutical drugs have infiltrated tap water, rivers and oceans around the world. A conglomeration of chemical insecticides, herbicides, artificial flavorings, colorings, antibiotics and even steroids taint the food supply. In addition, mainstream medical interventions—including antibiotics, antihistamines, amphetamines (for learning disorders), and the current average of 36 vaccinations per child—obstruct and impinge upon the proper development of a child's body, mind and immune system. Infants and children are particularly susceptible to the onslaught of these stressors because their immune, hormonal, brain and detoxification systems are still "under construction" and are fragile.

The stunning increase in primary childhood disorders during recent years *must* galvanize all parents into action. It is absolutely crucial that you, the parent, learn to protect your children from anything that can obstruct or compromise their health, while supporting and improving their health from within. This is the goal of **Natural Baby—Healthy Child**, which provides you with all of the information and insight you need to conceive and raise a healthy child in today's world.

Natural Baby—Healthy Child is organized as follows: The first three chapters identify and document the dietary and environmental causes of the worldwide decline in children's health, and offer solutions. These solutions include specific dietary choices, nutritional supplementation, environmental detoxification and holistic modalities.

Next comes a chapter on medical approaches, offering detailed explanations of allopathic (Western) medicine, naturopathy, homeopathy, osteopathy, chiropractic and acupuncture, including the pros and cons of each and how to apply the best from each.

This is followed by an entire chapter devoted to vaccinations, offering a practical explanation of their purpose, how they work and potentially detrimental consequences. After reading this chapter, you will be in a much better position to decide whether to give your child the standard vaccinations according to the standard schedule, allow only certain vaccinations (perhaps individually or spaced further apart), or approve of no vaccinations at all, relying on alternative ways to help your child's immune system develop to its full potential. This chapter also shows you how to administer homeopathic and nutritional support before and after each vaccination to help your child's body handle this "immune invasion," if you do decide to vaccinate.

Next come several short, instructive chapters containing specific advice on how to create and maintain optimum health during the various stages of your child's life. They begin with pre-conception and continue through nursing, infancy, toddlerhood and childhood. These are followed by a chapter on the maintenance of good health and the prevention of illness.

Appendix I is a treatment reference, arranged alphabetically, which lists specific medical treatments and remedies aimed at correcting the underlying origins of many common illnesses or conditions. These approaches can serve your child much better in the long run than pharmaceutical treatments that simply suppress superficial symptoms.

Finally, Appendix II offers a detailed explanation of common vaccines, with an individual appraisal and risk rating for each one.

During the past twenty years, I have helped pioneer the field of holistic pediatrics and earned a reputation as the leading homeopathic pediatrician for children in the Los Angeles area. I am a doctor of naturopathic medicine with licenses and doctorates in homeopathic medicine and Chinese medicine (including acupuncture and herbology). In 1988, I opened my medical clinic in Santa Monica, California as a general practice that utilized acupuncture, herbs, nutrition and homeopathy. Then, as my patients began to experience restored and robust health, they started bringing their infants and children to see me. Local M.D. pediatricians started referring their young patients to me when they were unable to achieve results with standard pharmaceutical approaches favored by allopathic medicine.

My goal for the past two decades has been unwavering: to find out what causes ill-health in children and learn how to prevent, treat and cure ill-health in the safest, most effective manner. **Natural Baby—Healthy Child** is the sum total of my training, knowledge and years of experience in holistic pediatrics.

It is my fervent hope that you will allow me to assist you in creating full and vital health for your children so they can live lives brimming with potential and opportunity, rather than burdened by sickness and disability. **Natural Baby—Healthy Child** is essentially a medical map that can help you keep your child firmly on the path to robust good health and the realization of the full potential of body, mind and soul.

Chapter 1

Dietary Problems and Solutions

Over the last one hundred years, the world has seen dramatic changes in the foods, dietary choices and the ways that people eat in the most "developed" countries, as well as in those that are "fast developing." These changes began in the early 1900s with the advent of food chemistry (the use of chemicals and technology to alter the structure of foods to preserve and extend shelf life). Around the same time, sugar in the diet began to increase, and today, the average person's annual sugar intake is 100 percent greater than it was a century ago, with an average of 22 teaspoons per day per person being consumed in America.[1, 2]

HOW OUR FOOD SUPPLY HAS DAMAGED OUR CHILDREN

The overload of chemical additives and sugar in today's food supply has greatly decreased the nutrient value of the foods we eat, while simultaneously imposing an ever-increasing toxic burden.

Children, with their vulnerable, growing bodies, are suffering the most. Remember: during infancy and childhood, bodies are still "under construction." Not only do those bodies need to take in sufficient nutrients for energy and maintenance, they also need them for growth. The quality, cleanliness and purity of a child's food and diet are critical.

Unfortunately, the health and nutritional practices of most of today's children are nothing short of abominable. Just look at these worldwide statistics regarding children's health:

- In the United States, childhood obesity has more than tripled in the last three decades. An estimated 20-30 percent of U.S. children are now overweight or obese. These children are developing elevated cholesterol, high blood pressure and type 2 (adult-onset) diabetes at increasingly epidemic rates.[3, 4]

- In the most recent study tracking the blood pressure of American children from 1988 to 2000, researchers concluded that the continuing increase means "that in another ten to twenty years we will be facing much higher rates of hypertension, heart disease and stroke as these children become adults."[5]

- In the Western world, including America, England, Europe and Australia, there has been an annual tenfold increase in type 2 diabetes in children over the past 15 years. It is estimated that one in ten children will develop diabetes in the coming years.[6]

- Even in New Zealand, where there is a rich history of raising children with a healthy, active, outdoors lifestyle and clean, nutritious foods, the government has noted that "an epidemic of obesity threatens to undo the significant progress made in enjoying our health and quality of life. Unless something changes, the current generation of young New Zealanders may very well be the first to die at a younger age than their parents." A four-year, $67-million anti-obesity campaign has recently been launched to raise awareness and encourage corrective actions.[7]

The sad truth is that too many of today's children are developing chronic health problems that will sentence them to lives of compromised health, potential, enjoyment and evolution. This means sickness, sadness and struggle, instead of health, enjoyment and vitality.

Fortunately, all of these ailments and conditions can be prevented, treated and reversed by improving dietary and lifestyle choices and exercising on a regular basis. But before we discuss the changes that need to be made, let's take a closer look at what food chemistry and an over-abundance of sugar have done to our diets and our health—and especially, the health of our children.

Food Chemistry

Chemicals were initially introduced into our food supply to preserve and extend the shelf life of foods. And once they found their way in, there was no turning back. Chemicals and chemical additives were soon added for additional flavor and color, a practice that introduced peculiar substances that had never before been ingested into the diet. Processing and refining techniques created food products that appeal to many people's taste buds, but have fewer nutrients. This food chemistry "wave" required an outlet for the mass distribution and sale of its products. Thus, the birth of a new food industry: fast food restaurants specializing in the preparation, marketing and sales of these peculiar, nutrient-deficient, chemically laden "foods."

Let's look at what a simple hamburger and fries from McDonald's has to offer to our children. According to the McDonald's company website, a hamburger consists of "100 percent Beef Patty, Regular Bun, Ketchup, Mustard, Pickle Slices, and Onions."[8] That itself does not sound alarming to the consumer.

However, if we then look closely at the ingredient list for this simple burger, we can see that the beef patty, which is labeled 100 percent Angus beef, is not organic. Therefore, the beef is likely derived from animals treated with hormones and antibiotics. It is further seasoned with a special "Angus Burger Seasoning" that contains 26 ingredients ranging from salt, dextrose, garlic powder to artificial flavors, corn syrup, caramel color (with known immunotoxicity effects) and partially hydrogenated cottonseed oil (containing trans fats, which are fats that have been chemically altered during the hydrogenation process, thus changing their normal structure and becoming a health hazard).

The bun that cuddles this "beef" patty is made with enriched flour, which is described as "bleached wheat flour, malted barley flour, niacin, reduced iron, thiamin mononitrate, riboflavin, and enzymes." It is then infused with high-fructose corn syrup, dough conditioners such as DATEM, and lots of artificial chemical preservatives. DATEM (Diacetyl Tartaric Ester of Monoglyceride) is an emulsifier primarily used in baking to strengthen the dough. Among its health effects are weight gain and possible kidney failure, hematological impairment, diarrhea, reproductive organ impairment, decrease of immune cells, increased urinary calcium secretion and thickening of the heart tissue.[9] Wow...that no longer sounds so delicious.

Then we add the French fries to the meal—primarily made from potatoes, but prepared in a vegetable oil that is a mix of canola, corn, soybean and hydrogenated soybean oil with added TBHQ and citric acid.[10] For the curious, TBHQ is a chemical preservative for oils that does not change color or flavor in high temperatures.

Many studies have shown that TBHQ is associated with carcinogenity and cancer, with lab animals developing stomach tumors and DNA damage.

Lastly, one cannot overlook the fact that these French fries are offered with ketchup, which is loaded with high-fructose corn syrup to reach the required sweetness that children have become accustomed to.

What are the effects of eating these hamburgers? An international study of 50,000 children published in June 2010 has shown that children who eat three or more hamburgers a week are immediately at higher risk of asthma and wheezing.

To add insult to injury, in addition to all of the chemical additives now found in the food supply we also find that many of today's foods do not contain the same amount of nutrients that they should or did in years gone by.

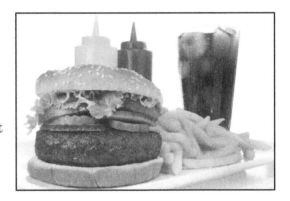

Factory Farming

The problem of nutrient depletion in our foods has been caused by the rise of industrialized farming. Fruits and vegetables grown naturally and organically by local farmers were replaced with "corporate farming" methods where crops are now "manufactured" rather than farmed.

When crops are grown, the minerals in the soil are absorbed by the plants, which use them to grow and flourish. Knowing this, farmers have traditionally rotated crops from field to field, and will let a field lie fallow for a season every so often so the soil can have time to re-mineralize and revitalize.

Following World War II, the pharmaceutical and chemical industries grew rapidly and became increasingly influential in agriculture and medicine.

In agriculture, for example, it was discovered that despite the fact that there are some 60 different minerals present in normal, healthy soil, most vegetables and fruits can be grown by applying just three minerals to the soil as fertilizer: sodium, phosphorus and potassium. While it's true that the presence of these three minerals alone will allow foods to grow, the foods will not have the same nutritional content as fruits, vegetables and grains grown in fully organic soil, which contains the whole spectrum of up to 60 minerals, along with a healthy population of bacteria, fungi, protozoa, nematodes and microarthropods that bring the soil to "life."

Genetically Modified Foods

The latest chapter in the continued perversion of the world's food supply by these "corporate farmers" is the use of the genetically modified organism (GMO). This involves taking a gene from one species (like a fish) and inserting it into the gene sequence of a completely different species (like a tomato) for the purpose of creating a fruit, vegetable or grain that is more resilient, less impacted by the environment and that behaves more like a machine than a living organism.

Obviously, these genetic mutations and splicings would never occur naturally, and they are described by many prominent scientists as playing "Russian roulette" with our most important commodity, our food. GMOs are unlike any other form of pollution ever created by humans, and we have no way of knowing what the long-term consequences of altering our food sources this way may be. When genes from one species are inserted into another species it is impossible to determine, control or predict what new and potentially deadly protein forms and structures will be created in the new genetically modified food. Our health, longevity and predisposition to different diseases as we age is determined and controlled primarily by the types and amounts of protein structures that we make and carry within us. With GMOs we are gambling with our protein structures. Proteins that have evolved naturally and extremely carefully over the past 100,000 years of human evolution to preserve our health and longevity can be interfered with, altered and turned in to the "Frankenstein" phenomenon overnight by GMOs.[11]

In April 2010 the Institute for Responsible Technology published the results of a two-year Russian study where three generations of hamsters were fed the same genetically modified (GM) soy that is produced on over 90 percent of the soy acreage in America. The hamsters and their offspring were fed their respective diets over a period of two years, during which time the researchers evaluated the health of three generations of hamsters.

First, they took 5 pairs of hamsters from each group, each of which produced about 7 to 8 litters, totaling about 140 animals.

Everything seemed to be okay for this first generation of hamsters; however, serious problems became apparent when they selected new pairs from the offspring. The first problem was that this second generation had a slower growth rate and reached their sexual maturity later than normal.

However, this second generation eventually generated another 39 litters:

- The no-soy control group had 52 pups

- The non-GM-soy group had 78 pups

- The GM-soy group had only 40 pups, of which 25 percent died

So these second-generation GM-soy-fed hamsters had a *fivefold higher infant mortality rate,* compared to the 5 percent normal death rate that was happening in the control groups.

But then an even bigger problem became apparent, because nearly all of the third-generation hamsters lost the ability to have babies altogether. Only a single third-generation female hamster gave birth to 16 pups, and of those, one-fifth died.

The results: nearly the entire third generation of GM soy eaters were sterile.

Unfortunately, avoiding food from GMO crops is not easy. Most conventional dairy products, as well as corn, soybeans, canola and cottonseed (the most commonly used vegetable oils), are often contaminated. And most conventional livestock products are now being raised on GMO foods.

Be aware of the potential dangers in GMO foods and consciously avoid them wherever you can.

The combined impact of corporate "factory farming" and "food chemistry additives" on the world's food supply has been nothing short of devastating. It has altered, adulterated and depleted the nutritional content of our most fundamental resource: the food and nutrients that keep us alive and healthy, and allow our children to grow and thrive.

Sugar

During the past century-and-a-half, there has been an exponential increase in the consumption of sugar by both children and adults. In the early 1900s, the average American man, woman or child consumed 83 pounds of sugar per year. By 1975, this figure had increased to 118 pounds a year, and today it has skyrocketed to an astounding 154 pounds of sugar per year. This amounts to 22 teaspoons of added sugar per person per day![12,13]

Plain white sugar (sucrose) and corn syrup are now ubiquitous in the food supply—they are found in processed foods, packaged foods, fast foods, junk foods, sodas, sweets, candies, chocolate, ice cream, condiments, sauces and many other products.

Before I continue, let me explain more about sucrose (white table sugar) and its effect on the body. Sucrose contains two components: glucose and fructose. Glucose is the form of sugar that our ten trillion cells require to create the energy they need to function. It is just as important to the body as oxygen and water. However, too much glucose in the blood can promote development of one or more of the "sugar disorders": mood disturbances accompanied by weight gain and/or obesity, which can then proceed into reactive hypoglycemia, insulin resistance, metabolic syndrome (aka Syndrome X), type 1 diabetes and type 2 diabetes. These illnesses can lead to a lifetime of symptoms, medications, restrictions and even cause an early demise, if corrective measures are not taken. (Each of these disorders is explained in the following pages.)

When a human being consumes sucrose, it is absorbed and then divided into molecules of glucose and fructose. Glucose is absorbed very quickly and creates a rapid rise in blood sugar levels. Sucrose contains high amounts of glucose and quickly increases blood sugar levels. Fructose, on the other hand, is absorbed more slowly and therefore does not stress or affect blood sugar levels in the same way.

The astronomical increase in the amount of sweeteners (sugar, sucrose, glucose, dextrose, maltose, high-fructose corn syrup, and so on) added to foods and drinks has led to the ongoing over-consumption of sugar on a worldwide basis. This has placed an overwhelming burden on the body's insulin production system, which is responsible for regulating and distributing glucose.

Effects of Long-Term Sugar Overload: The Sugar Disorders

When the over-consumption of sugar continues day in and day out, year after year, the body's ability to regulate blood glucose declines due to constantly overworking the production and receptivity of our insulin system. Ensuring that the right amount of glucose (neither too much nor too little) is delivered to the cells at the right time can make all the difference between health, vitality and longevity, or the development of disease.

Mood Disturbances

Whether children's mood and behavior is affected by sugar consumption in their diet has been a highly debated topic, and research articles and studies present different answers to this question. For the parent who wants to make the best decision, let's first examine the physiological effects of sugar on the body's chemistry.

Highly refined sugars and carbohydrates enter the bloodstream rapidly after being consumed (faster than the less processed counterparts like whole vegetables, fruits and grains would), and then produce extreme fluctuations in the blood glucose level. When blood glucose levels spike and fall rapidly, the body releases cortisol and adrenalin in response. These are hormonal steroids that are capable of changing body and brain chemistry, and which can then translate into symptoms such as shaking, sweating, increased movement and reactive behavior. Tantrums or aggressive behavior have also been noted in children.[14]

The most recent research on this subject demonstrates that this adrenalin release in children happens at a blood sugar level that would not be considered hypoglycemic (hence the different opinions on this subject), and it most often occurs around 3-4 hours after eating highly processed, high-sugar foods and drinks. This indicates that it doesn't take much for kids to "crash" into craziness shortly after a sugary snack or meal.

Setting and establishing healthy blood sugar levels in your child begins and ends with providing the right balance of proteins, carbohydrates, fats and oils at each and every meal. This always begins with the first meal of the day, our breakfast. There are numerous studies that show the importance of eating a well-balanced breakfast in the morning. Breakfast with a lower sugar load but more fiber and less-refined sugars and carbohydrates (such as oatmeal, bananas, shredded wheat, and whole grain bread) gives children a more stable blood sugar level with significantly smaller sugar crashes and adrenalin highs than the highly refined ones.[15] These carbohydrates should be served along with some form of protein (such as eggs, cheese or breakfast meats. Also include some form of healthy Omega 3 oil, such as flaxseed oil or cod liver oil, and you will give your children the perfect breakfast—an ideally balanced meal to establish and set their blood sugar for the whole day ahead, which will in turn allow them to pay better attention at school and improve short-term memory.[16]

Weight Gain

The Western and developing nations of this world are witnessing an ever-increasing epidemic of children who are overweight and becoming obese. The very latest numbers show that almost one in four children throughout the European Union, America, New Zealand and Australia are overweight or obese. As Professor Phillip James, chairman of the International Obesity Task Force, warns, "The epidemic appears to be accelerating out of control. Things are worse than our gloomiest prediction."

The reasons for this disastrous increase in weight gain are simple: too much sugar and refined carbohydrates, too much saturated fat and trans fats, and not enough physical exercise. A study from 2008 showed a direct correlation between the distance of the nearest fast-food restaurant to a school and the number of overweight and obese children attending that school. *The closer the fast-food restaurant, the greater the number of overweight and obese children in that school.* It is certainly no mystery. Hamburgers, French fries, pizza and sodas equal refined carbohydrates, which supply a massive sugar overload.

Obesity

Obesity is the medical classification given when a child goes beyond being overweight for his or her age and size. It is a medical diagnosis and condition that automatically increases the risk of a host of other symptoms and illnesses. It is also directly caused by the consumption of too much sugar and too much processed food. Childhood obesity has increased 400 percent worldwide over the past 30 years.[17,18] In the last 20 years, type 2 (adult-onset) diabetes began to strike American and European children for the first time in medical history. Type 2 diabetes is directly related to weight gain and obesity and, as the name implies, was previously diagnosed only in adults, who were usually over 40 years of age.[19]

High blood pressure, elevated cholesterol, reactive hypoglycemia and insulin resistance are also occurring in record numbers in children. If the obesity is not corrected, it will place an overwhelming workload on the heart, liver, kidneys and pancreas. Obesity is also the fastest destroyer of vitality and a child's self-confidence.

Weight gain in childhood is the beginning of a slippery slope of poor habits that can lead to a lifetime of poor health. Overweight and obese children are at an extremely high risk of becoming obese adults and of suffering from even more serious cases of the above-mentioned diseases.

It is not a mystery how obesity occurs: too much sugar, too much saturated and trans fat (from hydrogenated oils), too much nutrient-deficient food, too many chemical additives and not enough exercise and outdoor activity. However, there is also no mystery as to how to completely correct obesity: changing diet, improving lifestyle and getting more exercise.

The dietary habits and lifestyle choices that are established in childhood will become the predominant factors that determine your child's future food choices, exercise habits, physique and health. Obesity is a "lifestyle disorder" that can be reversed and corrected simply by following the recommendations outlined in this book.

Reactive Hypoglycemia

Reactive hypoglycemia is a condition in which blood glucose levels drop dramatically a few hours after eating a meal that is high in sugar or refined carbohydrates. The body's glucose-regulating system is overwhelmed by the sudden release of glucose into the bloodstream and overcompensates by releasing too much insulin, which lowers blood glucose to dysfunctional levels. This can cause an array of different symptoms including dizziness, nervousness, mood swings, irritability, fatigue, headaches and cravings for sweets and sugar.

Insulin Resistance and Metabolic Syndrome (aka Syndrome X)

These two glucose metabolism disorders have at their core a decrease in the ability of the body's cells to respond to insulin appropriately.

Insulin is distributed throughout our body and communicates with each individual cell via insulin receptors, which are situated on most of the cells in the body and are designed to regulate the amount of glucose that enters the cell. However, overuse or overexposure to glucose over a long a period of time wears out the insulin receptors. They become desensitized. **Insulin resistance** occurs when more and more insulin is required to "activate" the receptors and get the proper amount of glucose into the cell. Eventually, the body may not be able to produce enough insulin to do the job and the cells may "go hungry" or even "starve" because they can't get the proper amount of glucose.

Metabolic syndrome is a cluster of symptoms, including insulin resistance, that indicate the body can't metabolize and distribute glucose properly. Blood tests for a person with metabolic syndrome will show elevated fasting levels of glucose, levels that are high enough to be considered pre-diabetic, a decrease in HDL (good) cholesterol, an excess of LDL (bad) cholesterol, elevated blood fats (triglycerides) and uric acid. The syndrome can trigger a myriad of physical symptoms, which may include fatigue, sugar cravings, difficulty focusing and concentrating, constant hunger, low energy after meals, and body-wide aches and pains.

Both insulin resistance and metabolic syndrome may lead to diabetes if not addressed and corrected.

Type 1 Diabetes

Type 1 diabetes, for many years the main form of diabetes seen in children, is an autoimmune disease in which the child's own immune system attacks and destroys the insulin-producing cells in the pancreas. Lacking sufficient insulin, the body's cells are unable to absorb glucose. Symptoms of type 1 diabetes include excessive thirst, weight loss, fatigue, frequent urination, stomachaches, headaches and behavioral problems in children. The standard treatment is a lifetime of monitoring blood sugar levels coupled with the administration of insulin when necessary.

The majority of children who develop type 1 diabetes do not have any family history of diabetes, which indicates that genetics are not the primary cause of the disease. (Another clue is that there has been a worldwide increase of 300 percent in type 1 diabetes over the past 30 years. Genetic changes evolve much too slowly to allow for such a rapid increase to occur in only three decades.)

It is clear that outside forces are disrupting and distorting children's immune systems, and causing their own immune systems to attack their own pancreases. What could those outside forces be? Various chemicals, metals, insecticides and pharmaceuticals and vaccinations are all capable of provoking an autoimmune response in a child. Studies from around the world have shown a definite increase in type 1 diabetes since the introduction of the Hepatitis B vaccine. (In 1988 in New Zealand, the Hepatitis B vaccine was introduced, with infants receiving shots beginning at 6 weeks of age. Within three years, type 1 diabetes in New Zealand children had increased 60 percent.)[20]

Type 2 Diabetes

Type 1 diabetes is the primary form seen in children, but the seeds of type 2 diabetes can be sown in childhood through a combination of poor diet, excess sugar and fat, and too little exercise, resulting in the blood sugar mechanism becoming overwhelmed and failing at an early age. *Today, for the first time in medical history, type 2 diabetes is developing in children,* a direct result of poor dietary habits, lack of physical exercise and, in a stunning 85 percent of cases, obesity.[21]

Type 2 diabetes is characterized by consistently high blood glucose with fasting blood glucose levels of 126 mg/dl or more, or blood glucose levels of 200 mg/dl or greater, two hours after eating. These continually elevated levels of blood sugar create inflammatory problems throughout the body that can cause damage to the eyes, kidneys, brain and nerves.

Unlike type 1, type 2 diabetes does not necessarily require lifetime medication or dependence on insulin. It can be controlled and reversed by eating properly, maintaining a healthy body weight and exercising.

Toxins in Our Food

Most of today's food supply is contaminated with pesticides, particularly insecticides used to kill insects and bugs, and herbicides used to kill plants and weeds. In addition, a stunning number of foods contain artificial colorings, artificial flavorings, artificial sweeteners and preservatives, each of which are made from countless numbers of synthetic and harmful chemicals.[22]

Artificial food colorings, like the commonly seen yellow dye # 5 and red # 3, were originally made from coal-tar derivatives and now are synthesized from petroleum. Each one is a combination of several individual chemicals including benzenesulfonic acid, biphenyl and azobenzene.[23] Food flavorings are just as bad. A single imitation strawberry flavor contains the following ingredients: amyl acetate, amyl butyrate, amyl valerate, anethol, anisyl formate, benzyl acetate, benzyl isobutyrate, butyric acid, cinnamyl isobutyrate, cinnamyl valerate, cognac essential oil, diacetyl, dipropyl ketone, ethyl acetate, ethyl amyl ketone, ethyl butyrate, ethyl cinnamate, ethyl heptanoate, ethyl heptylate, ethyl lactate, ethyl methylphenylglycidate, ethyl nitrate, ethyl propionate, ethyl valerate, heliotropin, hydroxyphenyl-2-butanone (10 percent solution in alcohol), a-ionone, isobutyl anthranilate, isobutyl butyrate, lemon essential oil, maltol, 4-methylacetophenone, methyl anthranilate, methyl benzoate, methyl cinnamate, methyl heptine carbonate, methyl naphthyl ketone, methyl salicylate, mint essential oil, neroli essential oil, nerolin, neryl isobutyrate, orris butter, phenethyl alcohol, rose, rum ether, g-undecalactone, vanillin, and solvent.[24] Give your child a product that contains just *one* artificial flavoring and *one* artificial coloring, and he or she will be instantly consuming 30-50 chemicals that have never existed in nature, in the human body or in human history, until about fifty years ago, when they were first conjured up in a laboratory.[25, 26] If one artificial flavoring contains that many chemicals, think of the enormous numbers of chemicals found in foods that contain five, ten or even twenty artificial ingredients!

But that's not all: Hormones, antibiotics and steroids are now routinely fed to conventionally raised meats and poultry. Fish may contain mercury, PCBs, dioxins, antibiotics and many other pharmaceutical drugs that are now found in the world's rivers and oceans. Unless you're eating nothing but organic and locally grown fruits, vegetables and grains, it can be nearly impossible to avoid food toxins!

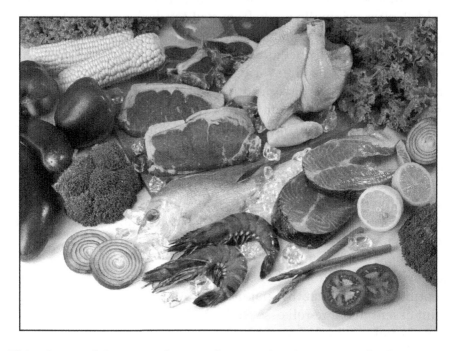

This chemical feast can have a devastating impact on the human body.

The chart on the opposite page summarizes the most common pollutants found in foods and their effects on the human body.

Always remember that when food is consumed, its ingredients are placed directly inside the body, where they will be quickly transported by the blood to all of the internal organs, including the liver, kidneys, brain and immune system. This is of particular concern to a mother-to-be, as everything she is exposed to has the potential to travel directly into the baby's body.

Pollutants	Effects/Consequences
Insecticides	Liver, kidney, reproductive and hormonal system abnormalities[27]
Herbicides	Eye, liver, kidney, spleen, intestinal problems; cardiovascular, reproductive and hormonal system damage; cancer[28]
Artificial colorings	Hyperactivity, brain damage, learning disorders, depression, asthma, skin irritation, hives[29]
Artificial flavorings	Hyperactivity, learning disorders, behavioral problems, lung and gastrointestinal damage[30]
Artificial sweeteners	Neurological and brain damage, depression, anxiety, insomnia, fatigue[31]
Artificial preservatives	Hyperactivity, neurological problems, cancer[32]
Antibiotics	Gastrointestinal damage, immune weakness, immune disorders, allergies[33, 34]
Hormones	Growth and developmental problems, reproductive system damage, hormonal abnormalities, cancer[35, 36]
Steroids	Early-onset puberty, hormonal system abnormalities, cancer[37, 38]
Mercury	Impaired neurological development, brain damage, mood and behavioral disorders, kidney and lung damage[39, 40]
PCBs	Immune, reproductive, nervous system and hormonal system damage; cancer[41, 42, 43]

Eating should reflect a conscious decision to give the body the sustenance it needs to sustain life. Food is meant to nourish us, create energy and help our brains and bodies function properly. It should also taste great and be an enjoyable part of each day. It should not contain foreign or toxic substances, chemical additives, metals or pharmaceutical drugs.

It's one thing to talk about the "shoulds" and "should nots" of a good diet, but quite another to translate these dictums into day-to-day living. Even with the best will in the world, most parents find that providing their children excellent or even adequate nutrition is much more difficult than it sounds. The dietary dilemma that parents face in today's world has two parts:

THE SOLUTION:
Providing your child with an exemplary diet

- *Diet alone doesn't provide sufficient nutrients*

  It has become increasingly difficult to acquire all of the necessary nutrients through diet alone because of the huge amount of processed, sugary, chemically laden foods in today's food supply. All of our children are exposed to these nutrient-poor fast foods or junk foods, and parents must confront this problem by setting serious limits. Even foods that are grown in the soil and eaten fresh or lightly cooked are not as nutrient rich as were the same foods in the past, because of the relatively poor quality of today's soil. As previously mentioned, the world's soils have become depleted through industrialized farming and increased population demands, which require fields to be in continual use, rather than letting them lie fallow on a regular basis.

Not surprisingly, foods grown in mineral-depleted soil have a lower mineral and vitamin nutrient content.

- *Exposure to toxicity and pollution raises nutrient requirements*

  Today, children in every major region of the world are exposed to enormous amounts of toxicity and pollution. This exposure increases the body's need for all of the essential nutrients, including vitamins, minerals, and essential fatty acids, to help neutralize and detoxify the environmental toxins. In short, it is more important now than ever for your child to receive the most nutritious foods available to provide all of the nutrients necessary for growth and development, as well as for protection from the terrible toxicity and pollution in the environment.

The Essential Nutrients

Healthy food is made up of protein, fat and carbohydrates (the macronutrients), which contain the subcategories of vitamins, minerals, glucose, fatty acids and amino acids (the micronutrients). These micronutrients are then digested and absorbed into the bloodstream and delivered to each individual cell. They are the building blocks for every tissue and organ in the body, and are necessary to produce energy, facilitate growth, development and ensure proper function.

Over the past fifty years these vitamins, minerals, fatty acids, and amino acids and other nutrients have been extensively studied. Some of them have been classified as "essential nutrients," by the National Academy of Natural Sciences , the most prestigious research institution in the United States.[44] A nutrient is dubbed "essential" only when medical research conclusively shows that it is absolutely necessary to one or more critical functions in the body. Essential nutrients must be ingested on a daily basis since the body can't manufacture them. When an essential nutrient is lacking, the proper development and function of body and brain will be compromised.

What Are the Essential Nutrients?
The "essential nutrients" include 14 vitamins, 21 minerals, 10 amino acids and 2 fatty acids.

Vitamins
A, B1, B2, B3, B5, B6, B12, folic acid, biotin, C, D, E, K, choline

Minerals
Calcium, magnesium, sodium, potassium, copper, iron, manganese, chromium, selenium, sulfur, iodine, fluorine, molybdenum, silicon, cobalt, tin, nickel, vanadium, phosphorous, chlorine, zinc

Amino Acids
Arginine, histidine, leucine, isoleucine, lysine, methionine, phenylalanine, threonine, tryptophan, valine

Fatty Acids
Omega-3: linoleic acid (found in fish oils and flaxseed oil)
Omega-6: linolenic acid (from evening primrose and blackcurrant oil)

For the recommended amounts of essential nutrients, see the chart on the opposite page.

Recommended Daily Intake Values for Infants and Children			
Vitamins	**Infant (6 months-1 year)**	**Less Than 4 Years of age**	**4 Years and Above**
Vit A (retinol palmitate)	1500 IU	2500 IU	5000 IU
Vit B1 (thiamin)	0.5 mg	0.7 mg	1.5 mg
Vit B2 (Riboflavin)	0.6 mg	0.8 mg	1.7 mg
Vit B3 (Niacin)	8 mg	9 mg	20 mg
Vit B5 (Pantothenic Acid)	3 mg	5 mg	10 mg
Vit B6	0.4 mg	0.7 mg	2 mg
Vit B12	2 mcg	3 mcg	6 mcg
Vit C (Ascorbic Acid)	35 mg	40 mg	60 mg
Vit D3 (Cholecalciferol)	400 IU	400 IU	400 IU
Vit E (d-alpha-tocopheryl)	5 IU	10 IU	30 IU
Biotin	50 mcg	150 mcg	300 mcg
Folate (Folic Acid)	100 mcg	200 mcg	400 mcg
Minerals			
Calcium	600 mg	800 mg	1000 mg
Magnesium	70 mg	200 mg	400 mg
Iodine	45 mcg	70 mcg	150 mcg
Zinc	5 mg	8 mg	15 mg
Iron	15 mg	10 mg	18 mg
Phosphorus	500 mg	800 mg	1000 mg
Selenium	*	30 mcg	70 mcg
Manganese	*	1.5 mg	2 mg
Chromium	*	*	120 mcg
Potassium	*	*	3500 mg
Inositol	*	*	*
Choline	*	*	*

Reference; U.S. Food and Drug Administration, Daily Values, April 2008

Healthy Meals and Snacks, Appropriate Proportions and Serving Sizes

So how do you ensure that your child is getting all of the essential nutrients, plus sufficient (but not too much) protein, carbohydrates, fats/oils and calories? The best way is to keep in mind the following perspective and picture.

The key principle in diet is balance: the right amount of each of the food groups in proportion to each other. Protein foods consist primarily of meats, poultry, fish, eggs, nuts and cheese. Carbohydrate foods are comprised of vegetables, fruits and grains like cereals, breads, rice and pasta. Fats and oils are found in meats and poultry (saturated fat), fish (omega-3 fatty acids) and vegetables, nuts and seeds (omega-3,-6 and -9 fatty acids).

The right proportions of proteins, to carbohydrates, to fats/oils at each meal is how you can ensure that your child does not consume too many calories. Imagine a plate and then divide it into 3 sections. Allocate 30 percent of the plate to protein (meat, poultry, fish, eggs), 30 percent to vegetables and 30 percent to grains (rice, pasta, bread). Dairy foods such as goat's milk or cow's milk, yogurt and cheese can also be included within the protein category. Cook with olive oil (omega-3 fatty acid) and incorporate flaxseed oil (another omega-3) into meals as a dressing for salads. Use butter (saturated fat) sparingly.

When your child eats a well-balanced meal of protein, carbohydrates and the right fats and oils, he or she will naturally feel full and satisfied. Children typically develop cravings for sweets, sugar and more unhealthy foods only when they consume excess carbohydrates, fast foods, junk foods and unbalanced meals.

Foods That Suit Your Child's Blood Type

As a homeopathic physician and pediatrician, I have had the opportunity over the past twenty years to study, test, and evaluate most, if not all, the different dietary guidelines and programs that currently exist. I have examined diets for both children and adults, including raw foods, vegan diets, various forms of vegetarianism, macrobiotic diets, low-carb diets, high-protein diets, the Atkins Diet, the Mediterranean Diet, the Zone Diet, the South Beach

Diet, the McDougall Program and the Dean Ornish Program. In my experience, each of these diets will suit a small percentage of the population for a small percentage of time, depending on each individual's particular health and state of mind. *But eventually, a person will need to move on to a sustainable diet that will suit them for the long term.*

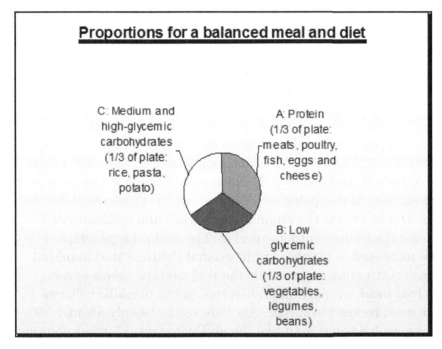

Proportions for a balanced meal and diet

C: Medium and high-glycemic carbohydrates (1/3 of plate: rice, pasta, potato)

A: Protein (1/3 of plate: meats, poultry, fish, eggs and cheese)

B: Low glycemic carbohydrates (1/3 of plate: vegetables, legumes, beans)

Each meal should also contain healthy omega 3 oils, such as olive and flaxseed oil.

What I have continually sought is an approach that works for all different types of people, all the time. The only system I have found that can do this is the "Blood Type Diet," which was developed by Dr. James D'Adamo. A naturopathic physician, D'Adamo first published his ideas in a book titled *One Man's Food is Someone Else's Poison* in 1980.[45] His system was then studied and refined, using lectin testing and coagulation studies to validate the theory, and in 1996 the results were presented in the book *Eat Right for Your Type* by D'Adamo's son, Dr. Peter D'Adamo.[46]

With this system and by understanding the differences between the four blood types we can then understand and appreciate exactly why it is that some people seek and flourish on a more vegetarian-oriented diet, while others require and prosper on a predominantly meat-protein-based diet.

The Blood Type Diet

The origins of the Blood Type Diet lay in Dr. James D'Adamo's research regarding the worldwide distribution of the four blood types (O, A, B and AB). O is the predominant blood type, followed by A, then B, and finally AB, which makes up only 4 percent of the population. Anthropological evidence led Dr. D'Adamo to conclude that O was among the original blood types and predominated during the hunter-gatherer period. The A blood type adapted and increased in numbers right around the time that mankind began cultivating crops, while the B blood type seems to have evolved most strongly and taken root in the nomadic cultures. The most recent blood type, AB, believed to be only about 1,500 years, evolved once man had the ability to travel farther distances, allowing B blood types to meet and mate with A blood types.[47]

The gist of the approach is this: for each of the four possible blood types there are specific foods that are more easily digested, assimilated and metabolized. Understanding which foods work best for a given blood type, and which foods increase wear and tear on the body, is essential to creating vibrant and long-term health. For example, many vegetarians scoff at the idea that anyone needs to eat meat. And there are meat eaters who think they would die if they ate nothing but vegetables. Why are the two groups different? According to the Blood Type Diet, type Os (46 percent of the world's population), do best on a red meat, protein-based diet, while type A's (40 percent of the world's population) do best on a more vegetarian diet with some poultry and fish, but no red meat. Viewed this way, you can begin to understand, appreciate and respect the differences in people's food preferences and requirements.

The principle behind the Blood Type Diet is that the foods that suit a person's blood type will be the easiest for his or her digestive system to digest and absorb, and for his or her immune system to handle. Why should blood type influence the way a person handles food? Each of the four blood types has slightly different-shaped antigen, or "antennae," situated on the outside of the red blood cells. These determine the blood type. And all foods naturally contain lectins—small, sticky, protein-like substances that will interact in a positive or negative way with each blood type. The size and shape of the lectins differs from food to food and will determine whether or not they will "fit into" and "stick" to a particular kind of antennae or blood type. *You don't want to eat the foods that contain lectins that will stick to the antigen/antennae on your particular blood type cells, because they can then compromise or block many important functions including digestion, metabolism, nutrient absorption and insulin utilization.*[48]

The Blood Type Diet can help you select the foods that are most effectively digested, metabolized and utilized by your child's body—as well as your own. It can also help you avoid the foods that put more stress and strain on the digestive, circulatory and immune systems. Utilizing the blood type approach to selecting the foods that best suit your child may also help you identify and avoid the foods that could cause allergies or sensitivities. In my clinical experience, 90 percent of the time this diet has improved allergy-related symptoms like skin rashes, eczema, constipation, increased susceptibility to congestion, coughs, ear infections and so on. And it has eliminated the need for further allergy testing.

Charts for each blood type

Charts for the various blood type diets can be found in Dr. D'Adamo's book *Eat Right 4 Your Type: The Individualized Diet Solution to Staying Healthy, Living Longer & Achieving Your Ideal Weight.*

Clean Nutrients From Pure and Natural Sources

Most M.D. pediatricians and allopathic medical associations still insist that it is not necessary to provide your infant or child with organic foods. They say there is not really that much difference between "regular" foods and organic foods, and organic foods don't bring about discernable improvement in a person's overall health. How can so many doctors be so poorly educated and uninformed?

Food is the very essence of what creates and sustains life. For at least 100,000 years, human beings have consumed pure, unrefined, unadulterated foods gathered and grown directly from nature. It is only during the past one hundred years that we've added insecticides and herbicides to our foods that are specifically designed to kill all manner of insects, weeds and microbes. Study after study is now showing that these chemical agents are capable of disrupting, injuring and harming the brain as well as the hormonal, immune and nervous systems of all human beings, especially babies, infants and children.[49]

A very recent study published in the *Journal of Pediatrics* (May 2010) conclusively linked children's Attention Deficit Disorder with the amount of pesticides found in their urine samples. The higher the pesticide amounts, the higher the incidence of ADD and ADHD.

Another study published in the *Journal of Pediatrics* (August 2010) shows the link between increased exposure to pesticides and the alarming trend of early puberty in American girls. This most recent study found 15 percent of the girls studied showed the beginnings of breast development at age seven. The average age of breast development was eleven years of age in 1991 *(Journal of Pediatrics,* 2009).

The herbicide atrazine, is one of the most commonly used herbicides through-out the world and has been shown to chemically "castrate" some male frogs and turn others into females able to lay eggs, according to a March 2010 study in the *Proceedings of the National Academy of Sciences.*

It is no longer a question of whether chemical insecticides and pesticides are capable of harming a developing baby and child. It is a matter of science and conclusive fact that these chemicals can interfere with and undermine both the development and functioning of an infant's and child's immune, hormonal and nervous systems.[50]

Organic versus conventionally grown foods

As mentioned earlier, the pharmaceutical industry started having a strong   influence on agricultural farming methods in the latter half of the 1900s. This included the introduction and application of insecticides and herbicides, as well as fertilizers. It was discovered that despite the fact that there are some sixty different minerals present in normal, healthy soil, most vegetables and fruits can be grown by applying just three minerals to the soil as fertilizer:

sodium, phosphorus and potassium. While it's true that the presence of these three minerals alone will allow crops to grow, the foods will not have the same nutritional content as fruits, vegetables and grains grown in fully organic soil.

The most comprehensive studies that clearly demonstrate the decline in the nutritional content in the foods that we are eating today as a result of these changes in agriculture and farming methods have been conducted by the American and English governments. The English government started testing and documenting mineral and nutrient levels in 20 commonly eaten fruits and vegetables in 1936, and the American government began doing the same in 1963. The table on the following page shows the results of these studies and how the nutritional content of 13 commonly eaten fruits and vegetables consumed in the United States, and 20 fruits and vegetables commonly eaten in Britain, has declined at an alarming rate over the course of several decades.[51]

Organic Foods and Nutritional Content

In normal, healthy soil there are up to four billion microorganisms co-existing in an active micro-ecosystem consisting of soil bacteria, worms and other creatures that are constantly enriching, oxygenating and transforming the soil into a nutrient-rich and mineral-rich matrix.

When crops are grown, the minerals in the soil are absorbed by the plants, which use them to grow and flourish. As mentioned above, knowing this, farmers have traditionally rotated crops from field to field, and will let a field lie fallow for a season every so often so that the soil can have time to re-mineralize and revitalize. It is the full complement of minerals present in healthy soil that gives vegetables and fruit their fullest and truest taste.

How many times have you been disappointed by the lack of taste in what looked like a normal apple, orange or tomato? This is due to the fact that it was grown in mineral-deficient soil. Lack of minerals produces lackluster foods that look good but do not contain what they should, do not taste like they should and do not provide all the nutrition that they should. Table 5 shows the mean percent difference in nutrient content between organic foods and conventionally grown foods in terms of the five most studied vegetables.[52]

Percentage Decline in Mineral Content of U.S. and British Crops in the Last Sixty Years		
Minerals	U.S. 1963-1992 (13 fruits & vegetables) in %	Britain 1936-1987 (20 fruits & vegetables) in %
Calcium	-29	-19
Magnesium	-21	-35
Sodium	N/A	-43
Potassium	-6	-14
Phosphorus	-11	-6
Iron	-32	-22
Copper	N/A	-81

U.S. (Berginer, 1997) and British (Mayer, 1997) data.
N/A - not analyzed

The worst kind of diet

The worst kind of diet is made up of foods exposed to insecticides and herbicides known to cause a range of ailments, from birth defects to cancer, and grown on soils depleted of minerals.[53] Lacing the food with artificial coloring and flavoring to make up for what is missing just adds insult to injury. And that's what you find in the majority of the processed and packaged foods usually found on supermarket shelves. These are not normal foods. What's truly normal is to get sustenance from naturally grown, pesticide-free fruits, vegetables and grains, foods that mankind has been consuming for the past 100,000 years. *Have we lost so much common sense that we think we can consume radically altered foods that did not exist until a few decades ago without suffering ill effects?*

Differences in Nutritional Content Between Organic and Conventional Vegetables: Mean % Difference for Four Nutrients in Five Frequently Eaten Vegetables*				
Vegetable	Vitamin C	Iron	Magnesium	Phosphorus
Lettuce	17	17	29	14
Spinach	52	25	-13	14
Carrot	-6	12	69	13
Potato	22	21	5	0
Cabbage	43	41	40	22

* *Minus sign indicates difference (in negative) of nutrient content on conventional crop from organic crop. For example, Vitamin C is 17% more abundant in organic lettuce (conventional 100%, organic 117%). (Source: Worthington, V. 2001)*

There's no question that the chemicals in insecticides and herbicides have dangerously unhealthy effects. There's no question that infants and children are more vulnerable to these effects than adults. There's no question that the chemicals contained in artificial colorings, flavorings and preservatives can and will affect a child's mood, behavior and actions. And there's no question that these chemicals can and will compromise a child's immune and hormonal system. This is a major reason why today's children are sicker than the children of just twenty years ago.[54]

A much better choice

Organically grown foods, by definition, do not contain any added chemical pesticides or additives. They come from organic, fully mineralized soil and will usually contain a higher nutritional content than conventionally grown fruits and vegetables. I will go so far as to say that providing organic foods is the *only* way to ensure that your child's health is not obstructed by foods as he or she grows, develops and matures. By carefully reading labels, shopping at health food stores and buying organic produce and meats, you can protect your child from foreign, harmful substances that have no right to be in the foods that he or she eats.

Avoiding Pesticides, Herbicides, and Chemical Additives

It takes more awareness, more time and more care these days to keep these harmful substances out of your child's food and diet. Although it is probably impossible to avoid these substances completely, the more you can avoid, the better off your child will be. When shopping for food, keep the following tips in mind.

Meat and Poultry

If you serve meat and poultry, always try to ensure that it's organic. Non-organic meats and poultry may contain steroids, growth hormones and antibiotics.

Fish

Look for wild fish from the cleanest areas and oceans of the world (Alaska, Hawaii, New Zealand, Chile). All "farmed" fish, unless organically certified, should be avoided, as they contain high levels of mercury and other chemicals from the food they are fed. These fish may also contain antibiotics. Generally, farmed fish are unhealthier than wild ocean-caught fish due to overcrowded conditions and disease transfer, which leads to the practice of routinely feeding antibiotics to farm-raised fish to control their infection rates.[55]

Milk, Cheese, Yogurt, Eggs and Nuts

Buy the organic versions of these foods from your local farmer's market or health food store. Non-organic milk, cheese and eggs may contain antibiotic residue and growth hormones.

Vegetables

Buy organic vegetables that are locally grown and sourced, whenever possible. Vegetables grown conventionally may accumulate pesticide residue. Typically the non-organic vegetables with the highest pesticide levels are sweet bell peppers, celery, lettuce, spinach, potatoes, carrots, green beans, cucumbers and cauliflower. The vegetables with the lowest amount of pesticide residue are onions, avocado, sweet corn, sweet peas, asparagus, cabbage and broccoli.[56] Be aware that washing and/or peeling your produce may help reduce levels of some pesticides, but it will not eliminate them completely.

Successful Treatment

My son David, now 10 years old, experienced problems from birth. He was hard to breast feed, had colic, slept poorly and was hard to manage.

My name is Julia and I am David's mother. Nothing in the world could have prepared me for the frustration, desperation and insanity that I have endured with one beautiful and very much loved little boy.

I have been unable to work, shop, attend church, go to a restaurant, go on vacation or even drive my car with David. No babysitter, day care personnel or school would take care of my son because he was so hard to manage. I felt as though I had been incarcerated.

Diagnosed with borderline ADHD, the obvious choice for David was medication, namely Ritalin, according to his teachers and school principal. My choice was homeopathic medicine. Growing up in England, I was no stranger to holistic medicine. My father, a medic in World War II, always had a cure for ailments using herbs.

Many phone calls later we found Dr. Murray Clarke, who treated children with this disorder. David was 7 years old and we were in our fourth school by then. I didn't mind that Dr. Murray was 35 miles away and the drive involved heavy traffic, because by then I would have traveled to the moon for this little boy.

I woke up each morning dreading what the new day would bring in the life of David, how many phone calls would I get from school, would he grab my arm from the steering wheel or would he have a temper tantrum in a grocery store that would go on for hours.

With the diet modification, vitamin program and homeopathic remedy that Dr. Murray recommended, one could see the calm, happy and loving child emerge, taking over the impulsive, agitated, hyperactive, belligerent and bad-tempered boy. School calls diminished, temper tantrums stopped, school grades got better and his soccer career flourished.

About once a month—depending upon the stresses in David's life, his growth spurts or changes in his diet—I watch for any changes in his being such as decrease in appetite, change in disposition, hyper-ness, restlessness, verbal abuse, aggressive behavior or abnormal symptoms. We know that it is time for his monthly homeopathic remedy and visit to Dr. Murray. Other than this life is normal…Thanks, Murray. —Julia

Fruit

Buy organic fruit that is locally grown and is in season, whenever possible. Conventionally grown fruit may accumulate pesticide residue. The fruits that typically have the highest amounts of pesticide residue are peaches, apples, nectarines, strawberries, cherries, grapes, pears, raspberries, plums and oranges. The fruits with the lowest amounts of pesticide residue are pineapples, mangoes, kiwis, bananas, papayas, blueberries and watermelons.[56]

Grains/Breads/Cereals

Buy organically grown grains, breads, cereals and pasta. These can usually be obtained from your local health food store, but even "regular" grocery stores are now beginning to include an organic section and offer a range of organic foods and products.

Supplements

Nutritional supplementation is a vital part of supporting and maintaining your child's health, preventing disease, and helping to quell or remove obstructions to health. Utilizing nutritional supplements can help ensure that your child receives all of the essential nutrients required for proper physical growth and development, and it also assists in the detoxification and elimination of the toxins that permeate our 21st century environment.

The following supplements should be given on a daily basis for 5 days of each week. (I usually recommend giving them on the weekdays, taking the weekends off.)

Multivitamin/Mineral

Your child's multivitamin/mineral formula should contain all fourteen of the essential vitamins, plus the primary minerals. These nutrients provide a foundation for growth while also providing antioxidants (vitamins that support the immune system), and also help to detoxify environmental pollutants that find their way into the body.

Studies continue to show that children who receive a daily multivitamin/mineral are healthier than those who don't. These children don't catch colds, flu or other infections as easily or as often.[57] They also display improved learning abilities, reading speed, mathematic scores and learning capacity.[58]

In a 2008 study reported in the *British Journal of Nutrition*, eighty children participated in a randomized, double-blind, placebo-controlled, parallel group investigation to assess the result of twelve weeks' supplementation with a multivitamin/mineral. The researchers reported that "Daily supplements of multivitamins and minerals improves the brain function of children with supplementation found to boost their attention scores and this represents the first observation of acute behavioral effects of vitamins and minerals in human subjects."

It is clear that the right nutrients can help your child's body and brain function beautifully and attain its full potential, just as nature intended.

An example of a high-quality multivitamin/mineral supplement label is on the following page

ChildLife uses only the highest-quality ingredients. Gluten and Casein free. Contains no artificial colorings, no artificial flavorings, no artificial sweeteners. Contains no milk, eggs, fish, shellfish, peanuts, tree nuts, wheat, corn, yeast or alcohol.

(Childlife Multi Vitamin/ Mineral supplement facts; www.childlife.net)

Supplement Facts

Serving Size: 2 Teaspoons (10ml)
Serving Per Container: 24

Amount Per Serving		% D.V. under 4 yrs	% D.V. 4 yr+
Calories	20		
Total Carbohydrate	5		1%†
Sugars	5g	†	†
Vitamin A (retinol palmitate)	850 IU	70%	35%
Vitamin A (beta carotene)	850 IU	70%	35%
Vitamin C (ascorbic acid)	135 mg	170%	165%
Vitamin D3 (cholecalciferol)	275 IU	70%	65%
Vitamin E (d-alpha-tocopheryl acetate)	20 IU	100%	65%
Thiamin (thiamin hcl) (B1)	2 mg	140%	135%
Riboflavin (ribo-5-phosphate) (B2)	2 mg	140%	120%
Niacin (niacinamide) (B3)	10 mg	100%	50%
Vitamin B6 (pyridoxine hcl)	2 mg	100%	100%
Folate (folic acid)	135 mcg	130%	35%
Vitamin B12 (cyanocobalamin)	6 mcg	200%	100%
Biotin	65 mcg	45%	20%
Pantothenic Acid (d-pantothenol) (B5)	7 mg	70%	65%
Calcium (lactate)	55 mg	8%	5%
Iodine (potassium iodine)	50 mcg	70%	30%
Magnesium (lactate)	15 mg	12%	3%
Zinc (gluconate)	5 mg	60%	30%
Selenium (selenomethionine)	35 mcg	110%	50%
Manganese (gluconate)	1.5 mg	100%	70%
Chromium (polynicotinate)	7 mcg	25%	5%
Potassium (citrate)	14 mg	*	*
Inositol	20 mg	*	*
Choline (bitartrate)	20 mg	*	*

†Percent Daily Values are based on a 2000 calorie diet.
*Daily Value not established

Other ingredients: Purified Water, Fructose, Lecithin, Xanthan, Citric Acid, Natural Flavor, Potassium Sorbate, grapefruit seed extract. Contains soy.

The above "supplement facts" box, required by federal law, gives a good example of the ingredients, amounts and serving dosage that should be found in a high-quality children's multivitamin/ mineral. A supplement label should also clearly state what other ingredients are in the formula and what is not in the formula (i.e., that it contains no artificial colorings, no artificial flavorings and no artificial sweeteners).

Supplementation with a multivitamin/mineral can begin when your child starts eating solid foods. If you are still breastfeeding when your child starts on solid foods and you are taking a good-quality multivitamin/mineral supplement, you can wait until you stop nursing before beginning to give a multivitamin/mineral supplement.

Cod Liver Oil

Cod liver oil is an excellent source of omega-3 fatty acids, which are also required for optimal brain function. While vitamins and minerals help improve how your child's brain functions, the omega-3 oils directly provide the key nutrients to support the actual physical growth and development of your child's brain.[59] 60 percent of the brain is comprised of fats and oils, and half of these fats are comprised of the omega-3 fatty acid DHA (docosahexanoic acid).[60] This makes DHA the most prevalent and important nutrient within the human brain.

Cod liver oil is the food and dietary supplement that contains the healthiest amounts of DHA, as well as large amounts of naturally occurring vitamin A, vitamin D and another omega-3 fatty acid known as EPA (eicosapentaenoic acid). For all of these reasons, cod liver oil is the perfect nutritional supplement for every growing child. Recent research has confirmed the wisdom of generations of parents in different cultures and countries who have given their children cod liver oil. Supplementation with cod liver oil during pregnancy and then while nursing has been shown to increase a child's IQ (intelligence quotient) by enhancing brain growth, size and function.[61] Amazing...including the right nutritional supplements in your child's diet can improve his or her IQ. So simple, so easy and yet, so profound.

You can begin supplementing your child's diet with cod liver oil as soon as he or she starts eating solid foods. If you are breastfeeding, be sure to supplement your own diet with cod liver oil. If you are still breastfeeding when your child starts solid foods, wait until you stop breastfeeding before giving cod liver oil.

Use only cod liver oil products that have been purified, tested and certified to be free of mercury, PCBs and dioxins. If this certification is not stated on the label, don't buy it.

Recommended Dosage:
For infants 6 months to 1 year: 1/2 teaspoon daily
For children 1-4 years: 1 teaspoon daily
For children 4-12 years: 1-2 teaspoons daily

Vitamin C

Vitamin C is the superstar vitamin for immune support, antioxidant function and detoxification of the body. Scientists began researching this vitamin in the 1940s[62] and since that time, it has been the focus of more studies than any other single vitamin. These studies have constantly confirmed that daily supplementation with vitamin C creates a healthier child.[63]

Giving your child vitamin C daily—in addition to what is found in the multivitamin—is like buying an insurance policy for his or her immune system. You will most likely find that your child will not get sick or develop infections as often, and will recover more easily and quickly if they do catch a cold, cough, flu, upper respiratory infection or ear infection.[64]

Supplementation can begin when your child starts eating solid foods. If you are still breastfeeding when your child starts solid foods, wait until you stop nursing before supplementing with vitamin C.

Recommended Dosage:
For infants 6 months to 1 year: 100mg daily
For children 1-4 years: 250mg daily
For children 5-12 years: 500mg daily

Probiotics

Probiotics, also known as the "friendly" bacteria, are good bacteria that are normally present in the intestinal system and are essential to the maintenance of a healthy digestive and immune system.[65] Probiotics help metabolize and absorb vitamins and minerals as well as protect against problematic bacteria, yeast and parasites in the small and large intestines.[66]

Lactobacillus acidophilus, Bifidobacterium bifidum and *Bifidobacterium longum* are the most important "friendly" bacterial species for children. For health maintenance and disease prevention, give your child a supplement that contains each of these species two to three times weekly. They can easily be added in powdered form to your child's formula, favorite drink or food. Supplementation can begin when your child starts eating solid foods and is no longer breastfeeding.

THE EXEMPLARY DIET: In a Nutshell

To summarize, you can give your child the best possible nutritional start in life by:

1. Providing clean nutrients from pure and natural sources

2. Avoiding pesticides, herbicides and chemical additives, including artificial colorings, artificial flavorings, artificial preservatives and trans fatty acids, whenever possible

3. Serving regular meals and snacks with appropriate serving sizes and proportions. For each meal maintain the optimum balance of protein (40 percent), vegetables (30 percent) and grains (30 percent)

4. Incorporate healthy omega-3 fatty acids into the diet by using olive oil for cooking, flaxseed oil for salad dressings and supplementing with cod liver oil

5. Providing foods that suit your child's blood type

6. Giving the right supplements, which include a multivitamin/mineral, cod liver oil, vitamin C and probiotics

Questions to ask yourself

I have found from my clinical experience and years as a homeopathic pediatrician that four important questions need to be addressed to ensure that your child is receiving the very best from his or her foods and diet. Answer the following to the best of your ability:

1. Is my child receiving all the "essential" nutrients (the 14 vitamins, 21 minerals, 10 amino acids and 2 essential fatty acids)?

Your child will receive all of the essential nutrients if he or she

- eats foods from each food group (fish/poultry/meats, dairy, vegetables, fruit and grains)

- eats many different-colored fruits and vegetables (different colors mean they contain different nutrients)

- takes a good multivitamin/mineral formula, cod liver oil, extra vitamin C and probiotics.

2. Is my child's food free from substances that are unnecessary or can harm, interfere and obstruct with healthy development and growth?

While it's impossible to keep your child away from all chemical preservatives, artificial chemical flavorings and colorings, hormones, steroids, insecticides or herbicides, if you provide predominantly organic, locally grown, fresh, seasonal foods, you will be making an excellent start.

3. Is my child eating the ideal foods for his or her particular blood type?

Once you learn your child's blood type, and use the lists of the recommended foods for that blood type, you will be in a position to provide your child with the foods best suited to his or her digestion, metabolism and immune system.

4. Is my child consuming a balanced diet?

Each meal should contain almost equal proportions of protein, grains and vegetables. Ideally, 40 percent of the meal should be protein, 30 percent vegetables/fruits and 30 percent grains. Add healthy oils such as flax and olive oil, healthy snacks and plenty of clean, clean water.

If you can answer "yes" to all of the above questions, congratulations! You're doing an excellent job of providing superior nutrition for your child and a strong foundation for a lifetime of good health. If not, you know the areas that need a little work. Keep striving for excellent nutrition: it's well within your reach!

"The doctor of the future will give no medicine but will interest his patients in the care of the human frame, in diet and in the cause and prevention of disease."
— Thomas Edison, 1903

Chapter 2

Food Allergies and Gluten Sensitivity

Nearly one in ten American children under the age of three is known to be allergic to at least one food, and the number of children in the United States suffering from food allergies has increased 20 percent over the past ten years.[1]

A food allergy occurs when the immune system mistakenly identifies a specific food or food component as a harmful substance, a foreign invader, and initiates a sequence of immune events to fight off the offender. Because a food allergy triggers an immune reaction, the body, brain and nervous system can all become irritated, aggravated and inflamed if that food is being eaten on a continual basis. *Normally, an immune reaction is an occasional short-term event in response to a specific pathogen that the immune system locates, contains, destroys and then disposes of. When an immune reaction is constantly being triggered or provoked, things begin to go wrong.* Approximately 10 percent of children of all ages currently suffer from food allergies, a number that has steadily increased over the past 15 years.[2]

FOOD ALLERGIES

A food allergy is a misguided immune system "attack" triggered by a particular food, which can cause a myriad of possible symptoms in a child. These symptoms can range from mild congestion, excess mucus or skin rashes, to headaches, mood disturbances and brain disorders. A true food allergy can be diagnosed with a blood or skin test.

Causes of Food Allergies and Sensitivities

The term for a substance that sets off an allergy is **allergen.** The most common food allergens and the symptoms associated with both food allergies and food sensitivities are as follows:

- cow's milk

- eggs

- wheat

- soy

- fish

- shellfish

- peanuts

- artificial food colorings[3]

- gluten

The above foods and food additives account for nearly 90 percent of all food allergies in children.[4]

Symptoms of Food Allergies and Food Sensitivities

The symptoms of food allergies and sensitivities can affect almost any part of the body and may include

- asthma
- ADD
- ADHD
- autism
- constipation
- diarrhea
- eczema
- learning disorders
- mood disorders
- recurrent ear infections
- recurrent sinus infections
- skin rashes
- sleep disorders
- stomachaches
- urinary tract infections
- enuresis (urination at night in bed)

Any of these disorders/symptoms can be related to or accentuated by food allergies, although the allergy is usually not the sole cause. There is often an underlying dysfunction within the digestive system, which initially leads to the food allergy or makes it worse. Food allergies place an additional burden on your child's immune system, which can also result in an increased susceptibility to catching colds, coughs and flu.

While no one can tell definitively which symptoms will strike a particular child, as a general rule the organ system that is genetically most vulnerable will be most affected and most likely to exhibit symptoms. For example, a child with a family history of asthma will be more likely to exhibit asthmatic symptoms in response to an allergen rather than digestive problems.

EFFECTS OF FOOD ALLERGIES ON THE BRAIN

Food allergies can affect the brain, and consequently behavior, just as easily as they do other parts of the body. The following drawing illustrates just how much one child's thoughts, feelings and behavior was affected by his reaction to different foods.

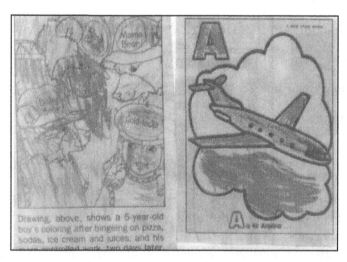

The drawing on the left shows a 5-year-old boy's coloring after eating pizza, soda, ice cream and juice. On the right is his more controlled work two days later after being placed on a diet of healthy foods.[5]

How do foods and food allergies affect the brain so profoundly? Because of the unique connection between the brain and the digestive system. Most people don't realize that before we developed the big brain in our heads that is characteristic of being human, we also had another brain situated in and around the digestive system. This brain still exists and is known today as the enteric nervous system. Wrapped around the digestive system, the enteric nervous system is a complete and fully functioning nervous system and brain unto itself.

Thanks to the exemplary work and research of Dr. Michael Gershon, who is known for rediscovering and defining this "original brain," we now know that nerve cells and neural pathways exist within the digestive system; the stomach, pancreas, small intestine and large intestine and the messages that originate there have a profound and body-wide influence on how we think, feel and act.[6]

To illustrate, consider serotonin, one of the brain's most important neurotransmitters. 95 percent of serotonin is manufactured by the intestines, where it can be found at all times. (Neurotransmitters are the substances that brain cells use to communicate with each other.) Every single kind of neurotransmitter that occurs in the human brain is also found within the nerve cells and "original brain" cells residing in and around the digestive organs. These nerve cells use the same substances to communicate with each other as does the brain in our head. *Anything that causes an irritation, inflammation or immune reaction in or around the digestive system can create a cascading inflammatory reaction anywhere in the body, including within the brain.* That's why what your child eats is so important. Everything that goes into his or her digestive system will have a direct effect on the "original brain," and an immediate secondary effect on the brain that resides in the head.

DIAGNOSING AND TREATING FOOD ALLERGIES AND SENSITIVITIES

If your child exhibits any of the symptoms of food allergies described above, you can take the following corrective measures, recommended in this order.

The Blood Type Diet

Begin by identifying your child's blood type and start feeding your child the proper foods according to the Blood Type Diet. In my 20 years of clinical experience, I have found that in 90 percent of infants and children with food allergies, eliminating the foods that do not suit the child's blood type will also eliminate the allergenic food and improve the overall situation. In the other 10 percent, following the blood type guidelines will help, but further specific allergy testing may be needed to identify the offending foods and the severity of the reaction.

Testing For Food Allergies

There are a number of different food allergy tests available through your health-care professional; unfortunately, none of them are 100 percent accurate. For example, most conventional allergy specialists utilize the skin testing method, which is usually reliable for a negative reaction (meaning it is accurate if there is no reaction to a certain food); however, a positive reaction (i.e., there is an allergy to that food) may be wrong up to 50 percent of the time.[7, 8]

Food allergy tests work by measuring a child's immunoglobulin reaction or response. Immunoglobulins (Ig), also known as *antibodies*, are proteins that play an essential role in the body's immune system. Their usual function is to attach themselves to foreign substances, such as harmful bacteria and viruses, and help to destroy them. In children and adults with allergies, the immunoglobulins react to certain foods as if they were foreign substances. They trigger the release of histamine and other inflammatory chemicals, which create the symptoms associated with food allergies. The main immunoglobulins involved in food allergy reactions are immunoglobulin E (IgE), which increases immediately after eating the allergic food, and immunoglobulin G (IgG), which increases in a delayed response to the allergic food.

Elimination and Detection with the Challenge Diet

This is the "home test" method, which can be conducted yourself. The elimination diet is a bland, low-allergen diet that does not include any of the foods in question. Provide your child with this diet for two weeks. After that, continue with the diet but introduce the suspected food in small amounts (1 tablespoon per meal) for a few days and note any changes. If symptoms arise at any time during the process, remove the food from the diet immediately. If no symptoms occur, increase the serving size for the next few days and continue until a full serving size of the suspected food has been given every day for a few weeks. If there are still no symptoms, start the process again with another food. It's important to introduce just one food at a time so you'll be able to pinpoint which food is causing the sensitivity or allergic reaction.

Skin Testing

Also known as the prick-puncture skin test, this method, which is still utilized by most medical doctors, involves puncturing the skin with a bifurcated needle or lancet and depositing a glycerinated extract of a specific food into the wound. Any skin reaction larger than 3mm indicates a positive response—an allergy. This test reflects immediate allergic reactions via the IgA immunoglobulin, which circulates primarily in the saliva, mucus membranes and skin. It is useful for testing the most predominant allergic foods, but as mentioned above, this test can be inaccurate by showing false positives up to 50 percent of the time. If this test is given I always recommend taking the ELISA test (see below) as well to give a more complete and comprehensive perspective.

ELISA (Enzyme-Linked Immunosorbent Assay) Test

There are two kinds of immune system reactions typically seen with food allergies: increases in the antibodies immunoglobulin E (IgE) with short-term immediate reactions, and increases in immunoglobulin G (IgG) with delayed long-term reactions. For the ELISA test, blood is drawn and food reactions are checked against both IgE and IgG antibodies. ELISA is my first choice of testing method, for it is able to detect both immediate and delayed food reactions, and can test up to 190 foods at one time from one blood draw.

RAST (Radioallergosorbent Test)

RAST, like ELISA, looks for evidence of immune system reaction in the blood, but it only checks for IgE antibodies. First developed in the 1970s, the original RAST has been replaced in most commercial laboratories with an updated version called CAP RAST or CAP FEIA. While RAST is an effective testing method, the ELISA test is preferable because it checks for both IgE and IgG antibodies at the same time.

Secretory IgA Test

This is the most recent development in food allergy testing and utilizes secretory IgA, which is an immunoglobulin found in saliva. This new technology has made it possible to test for IgA reactions against food by using saliva. All that is required is a saliva sample from your child. This is very helpful for testing infants and children, as opposed to the other tests, which all require the much more difficult and sometimes traumatic experience of a blood draw or multiple skin pricks.

Based on the results of your elimination/challenge test or laboratory food allergy test, you should reduce or eliminate any offending foods, while continuing to feed the foods that are recommended for your child's blood type. This is the best way to fine-tune the choices that will provide your child with those foods that suit his or her body, brain and immune system the best.

TESTING THE DIGESTIVE SYSTEM

Food allergies are usually both preceded and caused by a malfunctioning digestive system. In the majority of children with some form of food allergy, you will find that there is also some

---

Successful Treatment

Emily was diagnosed at six months of age with urinary reflux, a condition that makes a child very susceptible to urinary tract and kidney infections. At this time she was prescribed antibiotics to be taken daily on an ongoing basis to prevent these infections.

Over the course of the next year, Emily began to develop skin rashes, which were diagnosed as eczema, suffered from recurring yeast infections, had five ear infections over the course of eight months and caught almost every cold that went around her day care center..

The recurring yeast infections confirmed that the antibiotics had disrupted the balance of good bacteria in her intestinal and digestive system, a common side effect of antibiotic use, and which often leads to skin rashes and eczema. The recurrent ear infections and her susceptibility to catching

---

every cold that was going around indicated that her immune system had also been compromised and weakened by the ongoing use of antibiotics.

Obviously, her immune system was struggling and we had to find the right remedies to change this downward spiral and restore her immune system.

First, we adjusted her diet by placing her on the Blood Type Diet that suited her O blood type. By following her blood type food choices, we were helping her avoid the foods that she was most likely allergic to and that were irritating her immune system and aggravating her skin condition.

Emily was also started on her constitutional homeopathic remedy, Syc.Co 12 c, and nutritional supplements to support her immune and digestive systems: colostrum, probiotics, cod liver oil, vitamin C and vitamin D3, all of which are taken once daily.

After three months her parents began to see the changes and signs that her immune system was recovering and growing stronger again. No more yeast infections, indicating that the colostrum and probiotics had restored the digestive and intestinal system back to normal. Fewer colds and coughs, and she was recovering faster whenever she did start with any cold symptoms. The skin rashes and eczema were gradually going away.

It will take some time to bring Emily's whole system and being back to full health—probably at least a few years of taking the homeopathic remedy and nutritional supplements while continuing to watch her foods and diet. During this time the colds will become less frequent, her recovery time will continue to improve and her immune system will be able to protect her in the way that it was designed to do.

compromising condition within the digestive system. The digestive tract may be working poorly because it has not developed as it should or, more often, its proper function has been disrupted. In the latter case, the most likely suspect for causing problems within the intestinal tract is the use or overuse of antibiotics.

The digestive system is a very sophisticated and beautifully orchestrated ecosystem. Absorption of the nutrients from food is carried out primarily in the small intestine, with further processing in the large intestine, where the waste materials are made ready for elimination. In a normal, well-functioning and ecologically sound digestive system, all of these steps will occur smoothly. But if any of the organs, intestinal linings, enzymes, "friendly" bacteria or other components of the digestive system are compromised, digestive function will be impaired. The food will not be broken down efficiently into small digestible components, absorption of nutrients in the small intestine will not take place correctly, and elimination of waste products will not occur properly. Undigested and larger-than-normal proteins may then infiltrate the bloodstream and trigger an immune reaction or food allergy.

The following tests can accurately and easily help to identify any underlying problems in the gastrointestinal tract that may need to be addressed.

Stool Test

Just as important as the blood and skin tests that identify allergic foods are those tests that check the stool and urine to identify any underlying reasons for the allergy in the digestive system. A comprehensive stool test will identify imbalances in the ecology of the intestines and check for any of the following unwanted visitors/ conditions:

- dysbiosis (an imbalance or deficiency in the "friendly," normal, good bacteria that are present in a healthy digestive system)

- bacterial overgrowth and infections

- yeast overgrowth (most commonly, candida species)

- fungal infections

- parasitic infestations (most commonly found: clostridium difficile, giardia lamblia, entamoeba coli, endomilax nana, toxoplasma gondii, blastocystis hominis

An excellent lab for testing and evaluating intestinal function and stool analysis is Diagnos-Techs, Inc. which is located in Kent, Washington and can be found at www.diagnostechs.com .

Intestinal Permeability Test

Ask your physician for a urine test that checks for increased intestinal permeability (often referred to as a "leaky gut syndrome").

Increased permeability of the small intestine may develop over time as a result of ongoing irritation or inflammation within the intestinal tract. The "pores" or openings between the cells that form the intestinal lining become enlarged, allowing larger-than-normal food particles to slip from the intestine into the bloodstream, sparking an immune reaction. Decreased permeability (the opposite of "leaky gut") may also occur, a condition that inhibits full and proper absorption of nutrients.

The intestinal permeability test involves drinking a solution containing mannitol/lactulose, water-soluble sugars that our bodies cannot digest or use. The amounts of these substances eliminated via the urine can then be measured. Mannitol is easily absorbed by people who have a healthy gastrointestinal membrane, while lactulose (a larger molecule) is only slightly absorbed. Normal, healthy intestinal permeability will show high levels of mannitol and low levels of lactulose, while high levels of both indicates increased permeability ("leaky gut"). Low levels of both mannitol and lactulose indicates a malabsorption problem.

GLUTEN SENSITIVITY— AN EVER-INCREASING PROBLEM

Gluten is a protein found in all forms of wheat, matzo, couscous, semolina and other wheat-like grains which include; barley, rye, bulgur, kamut, spelt and triticale. Oats do not contain gluten; however, because they are always processed in the same mills, processing plants and grain elevators as wheat, barley and rye, this results in enough gluten contamination of oats that they can often trigger the same reaction. Companies who are aware of this contamination issue now provide oats that are processed separately and are certified on the label to be free of gluten.

Of all the possible food allergens and sensitivities, gluten is most likely to be the most prevalent and definitely the one that is capable of causing the most harm.

Gluten sensitivity occurs when there is an ongoing immune reaction to gluten in the diet, usually detected by testing for antibodies against a subprotein of gluten called gliadin. Until recently, blood tests were mostly used to detect these antibodies, with results indicating around 12 percent of the general American public suffering from this sensitivity. However, current research utilizing stool testing has revealed that these antibodies can be detected in the stool in up to 35 percent of the population. This means that potentially one in every three children may have this sensitivity and should be avoiding gluten.

Gluten sensitivity creates an inflammatory reaction. When these reactions cause visible damage to the mucosal lining of the intestines—which compromises the proper digestion, absorption and metabolism of food—the syndrome is called celiac sprue or celiac disease. However, when a child has a sensitivity to gluten, it is capable of causing an inflammatory reaction anywhere in the body, including the brain. Celiac disease is just one result of gluten sensitivity. There is a multitude of other symptoms and disorders that can be associated with or caused by gluten sensitivity:

- Asthma
- ADD/ADHD
- Autism
- Dermatitis
- Eczema
- Psoriasis
- Abdominal bloating or pain
- Constipation or diarrhea
- Gastroesophageal reflux/heartburn
- Inflammatory bowel disease
- Rheumatoid arthritis
- Autoimmune thyroid disease (Hashimoto's)
- Any autoimmune syndrome
- Psychiatric disorders

Testing for Gluten Sensitivity

Historically, the primary method for checking and testing for gluten sensitivity has been with blood tests that check for antibodies against gliadin, a component found within wheat gluten. Blood tests for gluten sensitivity continue to be recommended by most medical doctors. However, in recent years, it has been noted that not all children or adults who suffer from gluten sensitivity will test positive on the blood test. This is because the antibodies produced as the result of gluten sensitivity are mainly secreted into the intestine rather than the blood. This observation has led to the development of a far more effective and advanced method of testing for antigliadin antibodies through a stool test rather than in the blood. The lab that developed and specializes in this testing method is EnteroLab, which is located in Dallas, Texas and can be contacted at www.EnteroLab.com.

When to Test

If your child suffers from any of the conditions listed above, the first thing you should do is test to see if there is a gluten sensitivity that may be contributing to or directly causing the condition. If your child suffers from any type of autoimmune condition, or if there is a history of autoimmune disease anywhere in your family history, check your child for gluten sensitivity. This simple test can clarify for you whether this is an issue that you need to be aware of. You can dramatically change the course of your child's future health if you find that they are gluten sensitive and act accordingly.

When to Avoid Gluten

If testing confirms that your child is gluten sensitive, the only course of action is to avoid gluten at all times. Experience and research have shown that just a little gluten can create as much inflammation, immune reaction and harm as a lot of gluten.

Rice and buckwheat are the two primary grains that do not contain any gluten. Make rice your best friend and you will find that rice products can easily replace all of the foods that are commonly made from wheat, such as rice cereal, rice crackers, rice bread, and rice pasta. Rice becomes the grain of choice for gluten sensitive children and adults. Other grains that do not contain gluten are amaranth, corn, millet and quinoa. With the ever-increasing awareness of the number of individuals who are gluten sensitive, and the degree of symptoms that can be caused by this sensitivity, there are a number of food companies who are now making a wide array of excellent gluten-free products that you can find at your local health food store. Online, www.shoporganic.com also provides a good selection of organic, gluten-free products.

Successful Treatment

When Julia first came to my clinic at the age of 14, she already had a six-year history of ongoing stomachaches and constipation, for which her family had taken her to see many highly recommended doctors.

She had been given many different tests and prescribed many different medications including antacids, antibiotics, steroidal and non-steroidal anti-inflammatories, and had even been recommended antidepressants.

Testing by previous doctors included food allergy panels, stool analysis for parasites, yeast, bacterial imbalance and bacterial pathogens, an upper GI endoscopy and an abdominal CAT scan.

Now, six years later with no real improvement in her original symptoms of recurring stomach pain, she now also suffered from migraine headaches, fatigue and an underlying anxiety that was affecting every other part of her life-experience, including her social life and scholastic abilities.

Looking at this history of symptoms and the testing that had been done, I was extremely surprised to see that no one had looked or tested more closely for gluten sensitivity through stool testing rather than just the blood test.

After talking and listening to Julia to find the exact characteristics of her particular stomach aches, migraines, anxiety, fatigue and personality we prescribed her constitutional homeopathic remedy, Nux Moschata 6c, to be taken once daily and immediately ordered a gluten sensitivity stool test.

The gluten sensitivity test confirmed her sensitivity to gluten, and by placing Julia on a gluten-free diet and continuing to have her take her homeopathic remedy she immediately began to feel better. All of her symptoms began to

---

decrease in intensity and frequency and over the course of the first three months, she experienced 80 percent improvement, her self-confidence returned as her energy returned and she looked forward to school again. Her life had dramatically changed course.

HEALING THE DIGESTIVE SYSTEM

In addition to identifying and eliminating any offending foods and/or gluten and feeding your child according to his or her blood type, it's important to address and heal the digestive system and/or immune systems. This can be accomplished via the following methods:

Homeopathic Treatment

Consult with a well-qualified homeopathic physician who can prescribe the one correct homeopathic constitutional remedy that can enable your child's whole being to heal in the areas needed. Homeopathy is based on the principle of "like cures like," wherein the substance that creates the symptoms of a specific illness in a healthy person is used in a very diluted form to heal that disease in a sick person.

This principle has a documented history of understanding and application dating back to Hippocrates and was formed into a very precise method of medicine by Samuel Hahnemann, M.D. in 1810.

Nutritional Supplementation

The following supplements will help heal both the digestive and immune systems:

1. **Probiotics**—The three most important "friendly" bacteria for children are *Lactobacillus acidophilus, Bifidobacterium bifidum* and *Bifidobacterium longum.*

2. **Colostrum**—For most children, colostrum is very useful for improving and healing the digestive and immune systems. **Note:* If your child is allergic to cow's milk, *do not* give colostrum, as it usually contains small amounts of milk proteins.

3. **Cod liver oil** or **flaxseed oil**—Both of these omega-3 oils can help reduce inflammation within the digestive tract, while helping to re-establish and maintain the correct and healthy ecology.

4. **L-glutamine**—If intestinal permeability is a part of the problem, this amino acid is the most useful nutrient for healing and correcting the problem.

Dosages:

All of these supplements are available for children, with specific dosages listed on the bottle for different age groups. Follow the serving directions or consult with your health practitioner.

Osteopathic Treatment

Osteopathy is a complete system of medicine that applies a very sophisticated system of hands-on physical manipulation techniques known as osteopathic manipulative treatment (OMT). The exact spot where an obstruction lies must be discovered; then, the osteopath uses OMT to unblock and release it. Osteopathic treatments will always help to improve the function of your child's digestive and immune system by improving and facilitating the flow of your child's cerebrospinal fluid, lymphatic system and nervous system.

Particular attention should be given to the vagus nerve if there are digestive problems. The vagus nerve, also called the pneumogastric nerve, is the tenth of twelve paired cranial nerves. It is the only cranial nerve that starts in the brainstem and extends down below the head, running through the neck to the chest and into the abdomen, where it helps regulate the proper function and coordination of all the digestive organs. Consult with a well-qualified osteopathic practitioner.

IN A NUTSHELL

Food is the biggest and most important external influence on a child's health. The diet of the average child has changed drastically in the past thirty to forty years, and these changes have directly contributed to epidemic increases in the number of children suffering from ill-health. Poor food, poor diet and food allergies weaken the immune system and make a child more susceptible to colds, coughs, flu, ear infections, asthma and eczema. Food allergies and gluten sensitivity can also lead directly to mood and learning disorders.

To safeguard your child's heath, be vigilant about what he or she is eating! Provide organic foods, clean water and balanced meals, ensure that the digestive system is healthy and attend to any food allergies. The importance of nutrition, diet and digestive health simply cannot be overstated.

Chapter 3

Environmental Problems and Solutions

We are all exposed to pollutants and toxins from the food we eat, the air we breathe and the water and other liquids we drink. No living organism is immune to this. Even the Arctic and Antarctic regions—the least populated and most isolated areas of the world, with no industrial facilities—have experienced a measurable and considerable buildup of toxins and pollutants.

The native Inuit people living in the remotest parts of the Arctic wilderness have substantial blood levels of polychlorinated biphenyls, or PCBs, which are deadly chemicals used in industrial facilities as coolants, insulating fluids and electrical wiring coverings; dioxins, a group of highly toxic industrial byproducts; mercury from coal-fired power plants[1]; and brominated diphenyl ether (BDE), a chemical widely used in the manufacture of flame retardants and now known to be so harmful to human health that it has been completely banned from use in the European Union countries since 2001. Snow core samples from the Antarctic region reflect the increasing levels of lead that have been put into the world's atmosphere since the Industrial Revolution began, with the most rapid increase occurring when lead was first added to automobile fuel in the 1920s. The snow pack also documents the effects and worldwide pollution caused by the atomic bomb tests of the 1950s and 1960s. The most recent cause for alarm in the Antarctic is the measured and steady increase in persistent organic pollutants (POPs), which originate from insecticides and herbicides. Although these chemicals have never been in use in the Antarctic, they are carried there by the wind and the tides.[2]

THE PROBLEM

All of these chemicals and toxins have well-documented negative effects on the brain, immune system, hormonal system and, in particular, the growth and development of the fetus, infant and child.[3] If this toxic matter is accumulating in the least populated areas of the world, just think of what you and your baby are exposed to in highly populated urban areas! Some frightening facts:

- According to the American Lung Association, over half the population of the United States lives in areas that routinely have unhealthy levels of either ozone or particulate pollution (smog).[4]

- The United States Environmental Protection Agency (EPA) tracks about 650 toxic chemicals used in 23,600 U.S. facilities. The EPA reports that of the 4.24 billion pounds of these chemicals produced annually, about half is released into the air, ground or water. This includes chemicals from mining, smelting, power generation, paper production, electronic equipment manufacturing, plastics and pesticides.[5]

- A study conducted by the Mount Sinai School of Medicine in New York City found an average of 91 industrial compounds, pollutants and other chemicals in the blood and urine of nine volunteers who did *not* have jobs working with chemicals or live near industrial facilities. A total of 167 different chemicals were found in the group: 76 of these chemicals were carcinogenic, 94 were toxic to the brain and nervous system, and 79 could cause birth defects or abnormal development in children.[6]

- It has been verified that on any given day, almost 25 percent of the pollution and particulate matter in the skies above Los Angeles originated in China.[7] Air pollution is a *global* problem, with pollutants, toxins, chemicals, metals and even pharmaceutical drugs being distributed around the planet through the air, wind and ocean currents.

Exposure to this avalanche of environmental toxins is particularly dangerous for pregnant women and their unborn babies.

- In a landmark study published in the *Journal of Pediatrics* (August 2009), researchers conclusively linked air pollution exposure before birth with lower IQ scores in childhood. The children of the mothers exposed to the most pollution before birth scored on average four to five IQ points lower than children with less exposure.

- In the first study of its kind, conducted by the Environmental Working Group (an American-based research organization) in 2005, an average of 285 toxic pollutants were found in the umbilical cord blood of each newborn baby at the moment of birth. The blood samples came from babies born in U.S. hospitals in August and September of 2004. These pollutants and toxins included chemicals and metals known to cause cancer and damage to the nervous system and brain.[8]

- Recent studies from Russia show that a stunning 50 percent of Russian children are now born with some type of birth defect or physical developmental disorder, which researchers say is directly associated with the country's disastrous levels of environmental contamination.[9]

- The number of Chinese children with birth defects rose by 40 percent between 2001 and 2006, according to the National Population and Family Planning Commission. Birth defects are now the single biggest killer of infants on the mainland, with more than a million babies being born in China with "visible defects" every year.

- Forty years ago, one in fifty children in the United States suffered from some type of chronic, lifelong illness. That number is now one in five children, an increase of 400 percent. Exposure to environmental pollutants and toxins figure prominently in this extraordinary increase in sick children.[10]

This is the sad reality of children who are entering the world these days.

It is no longer up for debate whether exposure to and accumulation of toxins during pregnancy affects the health, development and intelligence of the baby. It is a fact. *Any environmental toxin that is present in the mother's body or that the mother may be exposed to during pregnancy can travel through her placenta directly into the developing baby.* As such, the only responsible action is to detoxify before conception, then neutralize exposure throughout pregnancy with vitamin C and other antioxidants.

For those who already have children, it is imperative to learn about environmental toxins, the harm they cause, how to limit exposure to them and how to protect ourselves and our children from their effects through neutralization and detoxification. These are the goals of this chapter.

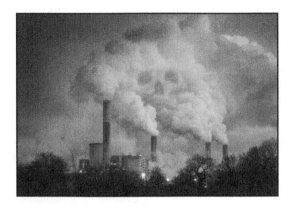

WHAT'S IN TODAY'S AIR?

Through our breath we are in continuous contact with the environment around us, and with every breath we take we inhale approximately a pint of atmosphere. Despite the Clean Air Act and other air quality regulations, nearly 100 million Americans are currently breathing hazardous and polluted air that does not meet the legal standards set by the Clean Air Act.[11] About half of the industrial emissions released into the air each year are cancer causing (carcinogenic) in nature. And, according to the International Agency for Research on Cancer, the air around industrialized cities typically contains a hundred different chemicals known to cause cancer in animals.

In the 1960s, burning trash in an incinerator was a popular practice, despite the fact that it released troubling amounts of toxic and carcinogenic pollutants, including a very potent one called dioxin. Even at just a few parts per trillion, dioxin is capable of altering biological processes; the EPA has since released a 3,000-page document concluding that the effects of dioxin on the immune system, reproduction and infant development are far more harmful than previously thought.[12]

Which pollutants are of primary concern in the air we breathe today? The following table summarizes those that are found in cities all over the world and their health-related consequences:

Commonly Found Contaminants in Today's Air	
Substance/Pollutant (from industrial facilities)	Effects/Consequences (on the human body)
Nitrogen dioxide	Respiratory illness, lung irritation and damage[13]
Sulfur dioxide	Breathing difficulties, respiratory illness[14]
Particulate matter	Lung damage, asthma, allergies, infection[15]
Polycyclic aromatic hydrocarbons (PAH)	Kidney, lung, bladder, skin, and liver damage; cancer[16]; chromosomal abnormalities in developing fetus
Lead	Brain and nervous system damage (especially for children), reduced IQ, learning disorders, behavioral disorders[17]
Ozone	Breathing difficulties, lung damage, asthma, allergies, reduced resistance to colds and other infections, reduced semen quality, infertility[18]
Dioxin	Immune system damage, disruption of the hormonal system, interference with reproduction and infant development, birth defects, cancer[19, 20]

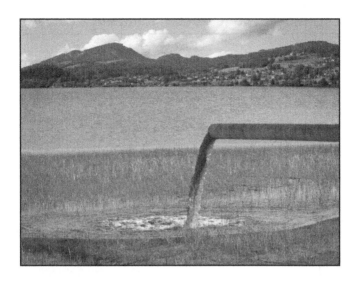

WHAT IS IN TODAY'S WATER?

Water is the gold, the currency of our bodies' matrix. The human body is approximately 75 percent water, its most dominant substance. Water is required by every cell in the body to deliver nutrients and carry away toxins. Water is the medium in which an unborn baby lives and grows within its mother's womb. Thus, it is vitally important for everyone (especially mothers-to-be) to use the cleanest, purest, most pristine water available for drinking, cooking and bathing.

Unfortunately, various contaminants (metals, minerals and petrochemicals) are found in drinking and tap water throughout the world. Although these contaminants are monitored and regulated in the United States, they still appear in the U.S. water supply. In other countries around the world, however, they may not even be regulated or monitored at all.

Commonly Found Contaminants in Tap Water	
Agent	Effects/Consequences
Inorganic Agents	
Asbestos	Cancer
Cadmium	Kidney disease
Chromium	Liver and kidney disease
Mercury	Kidney, brain and nervous system damage
Nitrites	Reduced oxygen in blood
Fluoride	Bone and teeth damage, decay
Lead	Brain and nerve damage
Copper	Gastrointestinal disease
Nickel	Heart damage
Cyanide	Nerve damage[21]
Volatile Organic Agents	
Benzene	Cancer
Carbon tetrachloride	Cancer
Vinyl chloride	Cancer[22]
Other Agents	
Aldicarb	Nervous system damage
Carbofuran	Nervous and reproductive system damage
Chlordane	Cancer
Heptachlor	Cancer
Lindane	Liver, kidney and immune system damage

Commonly Found Contaminants in Tap Water	
PCBs (polychlorinated biphenyls)	Cancer
Toluene	Liver, kidney and nerve disease
Xylenes	Liver, kidney and nerve disease[23, 24, 25]

Though the government monitors the level of pollutants in our water, that doesn't mean it's safe. Rather, all of these substances are still present in the municipal waters at so-called acceptable amounts, but the "acceptable" level of each substance is determined on an individual basis. No studies have evaluated the combined effects of continual exposure to all of these substances on humans, particularly children and unborn babies. However, the epidemic rise in childhood illnesses and learning disorders indicates that these substances are not as innocuous as the authorities may believe.

THE BIG GUNS—Today's most common contaminants

Approximately 70,000 chemicals are in use and have been detected throughout the world, with some 30,000 on the market today that have not been assessed for human health risk. Around 1,500 new chemicals are introduced each year. The majority of the chemicals in existence are manmade and did not exist 100 or even 60 years ago. Yet the human body evolved in an environment containing only naturally occurring organic substances over a period of at least 100,000 years. Our bodies are not designed or equipped to deal with constant or even intermittent exposure to toxic metals, harmful chemicals, cancer-causing substances and body-altering hormones, steroids and other pharmaceuticals. A child's body is even less capable and equipped to deal with these toxic substances because their immune, nervous and detoxification systems are still "under construction." Children, especially unborn babies, are extremely vulnerable to these hazardous chemicals, as evidenced by the increasing number born with brain damage from prenatal exposure.[26]

The most harmful chemicals, those with documented negative effects on children and the human body in general, which are also extremely prevalent in the environment, include the following:

The Most Harmful Chemicals in the Air, Water and Food	
Substance	Effects/ Consequences
Lead (metal) Most commonly found in lead based paint, soil, drinking water and air.	Nervous system and brain damage, learning and behavioral disorders, reproductive and hormonal system damage, reduced IQ[27]
Mercury (metal) Most commonly found in dental amalgams (40-50% mercury), fish, air and water.	Brain and nervous system damage and disorders, autism, kidney damage[28, 29]
Phthalates (plastics) Most commonly found in plastic toys, plastic food containers, food wrap, vinyl flooring, shower curtains, non-organic baby care products, indoor air.	Hormonal abnormalities and damage, liver, kidney and lung damage, decreased size and function of baby boy's testicles[30]
Bisphenol-A (plastics) Most commonly found in plastic baby and water bottles, canned foods, canned soft drinks.	Hormonal system disruption and disorders, cancer, nerve and developmental toxicity (brain damage)[31, 32]

The Most Harmful Chemicals in the Air, Water and Food	
Substance	Effects/ Consequences
PBDEs (fire retardants) Most commonly found in mattresses, pillows, blankets, upholstery, electronic equipment, indoor air.	Hormonal disorders, infertility, thyroid disorders, abnormal brain development, liver toxicity[33, 34]

Lead

Recent studies show that even very small amounts of lead can affect the brain's development during pregnancy and at any time throughout childhood, decreasing IQ by up to 10 points.[35] Recent U.S. studies have concluded that one-third of the cases of ADHD are linked to prenatal exposure to lead and cigarette smoke. Children found with blood lead concentrations of just 2 mcg/dL or more had four times the incidence of ADHD, compared to those with the lowest blood levels of lead.[36, 37] Yet, inexplicably, the Centers for Disease Control and Prevention (CDC) considers five times that amount (10 mcg/dL) to be safe.

This outdated safety standard for lead should be re-evaluated in today's world, with all the most recent studies demonstrating that babies and children are particularly and acutely sensitive and susceptible to very, very small amounts of this toxic material. The effect of lead on babies and children varies, depending on the individual predisposition, sensitivity and susceptibility of each child. This means that there really is no known level of exposure that is completely safe and acceptable.

Mercury

Around the world, approximately 50 percent of the mercury

released into the air and environment is from coal-fired power plants. Industrial boilers and heaters emit another 15 percent and cement manufacturing plants another 7 percent. This mercury then ends up in our soil, lakes, rivers and oceans. Mercury exposure and accumulation caused by eating fish has received a lot of attention and study around the world in recent years. We are also directly exposed to this toxic metal through the use of amalgam dental fillings, which contain up to 50 percent mercury, and yet continue to be placed in children's and adults' mouths by dentists around the world.[38] Studies now show that this metal is a problem for everybody, and is especially hazardous to the mother and developing baby. The United States Food and Drug Administration (FDA) has even gone to the extraordinary point of publishing which fish—based on mercury content—are okay to consume and how often they may be eaten safely by pregnant women and babies.[39] Some countries, including Sweden, have now passed legislation that regulates and restricts the use or application of mercury amalgam fillings in pregnant women and/or nursing mothers.[40]

Phthalates

In 2004, manufacturers worldwide produced more than 800 million pounds of phthalates, a group of chemical compounds used in the manufacturing of beauty products and plastics to make them soft and flexible. Ongoing tests document the presence and accumulation of these chemicals in children and adults throughout the United States. Phthalates particularly disrupt and interfere with the function and normal development of the hormonal system; studies now show conclusively that they can cause changes in the size and anatomy of the genitals of baby boys.[41] A recent report, published in the *Journal of Pediatrics* in February 2008, found that 80 percent of infants had at least seven different types of phthalates in their urine.[42] The use of phthalates is unregulated in the U.S., but in Europe they have been banned from use in all baby toys and cosmetics.[43] Canada is the most recent country to completely outlaw the use of phthalates.

Bisphenol-A (BPA)

Bisphenol-A is another chemical in widespread use and detected in nearly all humans tested in the United States. This chemical is also used in the manufacturing of plastics, particularly hard, clear polycarbonate plastics used for baby bottles, water bottles, and other food and beverage containers. This chemical leaches from the plastic, especially when the containers are heated or microwaved, cleaned with detergents or exposed to acidic foods and drinks. Of 115 studies examining low-dose exposure of this chemical, 94 found harmful effects, including decreased testosterone levels, enlarged prostates and lower sperm counts in newborn males, as well as early puberty and disrupted hormonal cycles in girls.[44]

Polybrominated diphenyl ethers (PBDEs)

PBDEs are chemicals used as fire retardants on many common household products, including mattresses, upholstery, blankets, fabrics and electronic equipment. Along with brominated diphenyl ethers (BDEs), PBDEs are in widespread use throughout the world. In an extensive Swedish study, scientists found that PBDEs accumulated within breast milk and other tissues, which means the chemical is being directly consumed by nursing babies. Studies show these chemicals interfere with normal brain development, alter sex hormones, reduce male fertility and disrupt ovary development.[31, 32, 35, 45]

In 2004, the European Union banned the use of PBDEs due to their recognition of the severe health hazards associated with this chemical.

Successful treatment

Paula was 15 years old when I saw her in 2007. She had a long history of migraine headaches. She had been prescribed pharmaceutical medications, which would sometimes help alleviate the pain and discomfort but never changed the ongoing pattern of recurring migraines. In addition, she also had difficulty sleeping, tending to wake during the night and have trouble getting back into a deep sleep.

She is a very sensitive person—sensitive to loud noises, perfumes and other chemical smells, the quality and taste of foods and other people's energy..

There can be many different reasons that contribute to the very painful symptom of migraine headaches. Looking at Paula's situation, we first tested and ruled out any food allergies or gluten sensitivity. Her regular blood chemistry, blood sugar and blood count panels were okay. To look more closely to see if there were any physical or external triggers that may be aggravating her migraines, we conducted a hair analysis and special urine test to measure the amount of metals in her system. These tests indicated an elevated amount of cadmium and mercury..

Paula talked about her life and how her saving grace and favorite passion had always been dancing, which she started at age 5. She also spoke of how the most difficult part of life for her had been her relationship with her father, who she described as quite mean and verbally abusive, "a bit of a monster."

Paula was prescribed the homeopathic remedy stramonium, starting with 9c, one pellet once daily, as her homeopathic constitutional remedy. In addition Paula was also prescribed HM Nano-Detox liquid and Vitamin C 1000mg daily to gently help her body detoxify and eliminate the accumulated cadmium and mercury.

It took three months of taking the homeopathic remedy and adjusting the dosage every six weeks along with the detox supplements before the migraines began to decrease in frequency and intensity. Over the course of the next year as Paula continued to take her remedy, her sleep improved and the migraines continued to decrease, and now she has not had a migraine for the past two years.

THE SOLUTION

First, we must acknowledge the reality of today's world. *Every year, in the United States alone, 4.24 billion pounds of toxic, carcinogenic and hormone-altering chemicals and metals are released into the environment. This is not going to stop or change dramatically in the foreseeable future.*

It is our demand for and dependence on the products created by industry— oil, electricity, appliances, containers, food, clothing, and so on—that has led to the creation of our toxic environment. *Regardless of who is to blame for the present state of our world, we must do what we can to improve things for ourselves and our children by limiting exposure to toxins, and neutralizing, detoxifying and eliminating as many of these substances as possible before they can cause internal harm.*

Limit Exposure to Toxins

Becoming aware of these pollutants and their effects on the human body is the first step toward reducing exposure for yourself and your family.

The next step is to take charge of your home environment. Ensure that all of these items are made from the safest, non-toxic materials and products available: carpets, wood floors, furniture, fabrics, paints, cooking and food storing containers, cleaning products, soaps, laundry detergents, air filtration systems, lawn care and pesticides. If you live within a city, a high-quality HEPA air filtration system is also highly recommended to improve and detoxify the air within your home.

Your choices will, in large part, determine the level of toxins in your home.

Most of the time, it is not possible to control our exposure to toxins in the external environment. That's why it is so important make sure your home is the safest, least toxic environment possible.

Identify Toxins in Your Body

You can identify the amount and kinds of harmful substances that have accumulated in your body via the following testing methods:

Metal Testing

Testing for lead, mercury, arsenic, cadmium, aluminum, nickel, tin and other metals is usually best accomplished through analysis of your hair and/or urine. There is a routine blood test for lead, but not for the other metals, and the amount of lead in the blood does not necessarily reflect the total amount of lead in the body. This is because lead travels from the lungs and intestinal tract to the blood and then is gradually removed from the blood and stored in tissues such as organs, bones and teeth. This is the body's response to most metals, which makes hair and urine samples more useful for determining the amount of exposure and accumulation of these toxins.

Chemical Testing

Samples may be taken of your blood, urine, breast milk, or even semen, to analyze levels of toxic chemicals. The laboratory that specializes in testing for environmental toxins in the U.S. is Metametrix Lab, which can be located at (www.metametrix.com).

Digestive and Intestinal Ecology and Function

This involves a comprehensive stool and digestive analysis (CDSA), which can evaluate your body's digestive function for proteins, fats and carbohydrates, intestinal permeability, intestinal ecology, and the presence of any unwanted bacterial, yeast, fungal or parasitic invaders.

Liver, Kidney Function and Blood Chemistry

A traditional comprehensive blood panel can determine your basic blood chemistry along with an analysis of the red blood cells, immune white blood cells and check for liver, kidney and thyroid function.

Evaluation and Priorities

Once you obtain this information via your naturopathic doctor, osteopathic doctor or holistically oriented M.D., you can zero in on areas or the types of toxins that require the most attention. A physician who is experienced in evaluating these tests can then prioritize the results and prescribe an effective detoxification program.

The beauty of testing is that you can retest to monitor the effectiveness of the detoxification and ensure that these substances have been successfully eliminated for future health, or prior to conception if you are planning to become pregnant.

You can work directly with a health professional who is well versed in detoxification methods to design a detox program specifically for you. Or you can use the following suggestions as a guide.

Neutralize, Detoxify and Eliminate Toxins

Detoxification involves capturing and neutralizing the pollutant or toxin and transporting it safely out of the body. The body has three primary methods for detoxifying and eliminating pollutants: methylation, sulfation and antioxidants. Antioxidants such as vitamin C, vitamin E and alpha lipoic acid, are capable of neutralizing toxins and assisting in their removal from the body. The liver utilizes the methods of methylation and sulfation to render toxins harmless enough that they can then be safely transferred and eliminated through the bile and intestinal tract, or through the kidneys and urine. The methylation pathway utilizes nutrients like TMG, DMG and SAMe (S-adenosyl-L-methionine) which are all are methyl donors that also help in the production of several brain chemicals and can improve mood, energy, alertness and concentration. Sulfation is achieved with MSM (methylsulfonylmethane) or sulfur-containing amino acids like methionine, cysteine and glutathione.

As mentioned above, various laboratory tests can identify the substances that may have accumulated in the body, including hair and urine analysis to detect metals, organic acid analysis of the urine to monitor chemicals, stool analysis to identify digestive and intestinal ecology, and a regular comprehensive blood panel to monitor blood chemistry with liver and kidney function. These tests will help you prioritize the toxins that require the most attention. Or you can follow the recommendations that follow, which will address the complete spectrum of metal, chemical, liver and intestinal detoxification.

Detoxify *Before* Conceiving

Before we get into the mechanics of detoxification, I must make an important point: Periodically detoxifying and cleansing the body is a great way to ensure good health, vitality and longevity.

Additionally, detoxifying prior to conception can be an important part of preparing your body for pregnancy. *However, detoxification should only be attempted before conceiving, not during the pregnancy.* Detoxification during pregnancy carries the risk of exposing the baby to higher levels of toxins.

Most toxins accumulate and are stored in body fat and connective tissues, which is the body's way of placing these potentially harmful substances into "isolation" and keeping them away from more vital organs like the brain. When you begin the process of detoxification, you'll dislodge and release these toxins into your bloodstream, lungs, liver and intestines so they can be eliminated. Thus, your levels of actively circulating toxins may temporarily increase on their way to being eliminated. Unfortunately, if you happen to be pregnant, your developing baby will be exposed to this release and onslaught of toxins. That's why it is always best to complete the detoxification process *prior* to conception and *not pursue it at all during pregnancy.*

The Great Detoxifier: The Liver

The liver is the primary organ of detoxification and is equipped with the following abilities for identifying, neutralizing and disposing of toxic substances.

Filtering the Blood

Every minute, approximately two quarts of blood pass through the liver for detoxification. During this stage, a healthy liver will be able to filter out over 90 percent of the toxins in the blood, most of which will then be combined with bile and excreted.

Bile Excretion

Each day, the liver produces approximately one quart of bile, which is used as a "transport vehicle" for carrying toxic substances into the intestines, where they will be eliminated through the stool.

Neutralizing Toxins (Phase I Detoxification)

A two-step enzymatic process within the liver converts toxic chemicals into less harmful substances that can be safely escorted out of the body. The liver accomplishes this through three main chemical reactions (oxidation, reduction and hydrolysis), plus the use of cytochrome P450 enzymes. The most important nutrients for supporting phase I detoxification are the antioxidants: vitamin C, vitamin E, selenium, glutathione and alpha-lipoic acid.

Making Toxins Water Soluble (Phase II Detoxification)

During this step, referred to as the conjugation pathway, the liver adds another substance to the toxin to make it less harmful and which also makes it water soluble so it can be excreted out of the body through bile or urine. Phase II detoxification is carried out by methylation and sulfation, as mentioned previously. The most important nutrients for phase II detoxification include cysteine, methionine, glycine, acetyl-CoA, MSM), SAMe) and glutathione.

The liver requires the right amounts of vitamins, minerals, amino acids and antioxidants to be able to effectively and continuously detoxify and protect the rest of the body and brain. You can assist the liver by taking the supplements that provide these specific nutrients.

Other Methods of Detoxification

Of course, taking supplements isn't the only way to support the liver. The general tenets of good health apply: eat a clean, healthful diet, get plenty of exercise, sleep, reduce your exposure to toxins, and so on. But a few recommendations may be particularly effective:

Consume Adequate Fiber

After the liver has processed and neutralized toxins, they are combined with bile and dumped into the intestines. By consuming plenty of fiber, you can help your body ferry these substances through the intestines and eliminate them with a minimum of reabsorption.

Drink Plenty of Water

Pure water is essential for the effective transportation and flushing of toxins from the body through the urine and feces after they have been processed by the liver.

The Sauna

The sauna is a wonderful and extremely effective method for helping the body detoxify and eliminate metals and chemicals. There are infra-red saunas and regular heated saunas, and some research indicates that infra-red has some extra detoxifying attributes. But essentially any sauna can be an effective part of a detoxification program.[46, 47]

Pre-Conception Detox Protocol

The following detoxification formulas and protocols are designed for both the mother-to-be and the father-to-be (the health and vitality of the father's sperm is just as important as the mother's health for determining and creating the foundation of health for the baby). Begin at least 3 months prior to conception and take these formulas 5 days per week, with 2 days off each week to allow the body to process and eliminate the toxins. Be sure to drink ample amounts of pure spring water (at least 4-6 glasses daily) throughout the process. Specific dosages will be noted on the product label.

1. Start with *ClearVite by Apex Energetics* for a systemic cleansing and detoxification effect on the digestive system, liver and kidneys.

   Key ingredients:

   - Silymarin (milk thistle)

   - N-acetyl-L-cysteine

   - L- glutamine

   - L-lysine

   - Glycine

   - Probiotics: Lactobacillus Acidophilus

   - Enzymes: amylase, cellulose, protease

2. After two weeks, you are ready to work more deeply, to detoxify and   eliminate metals and additional chemicals by adding

   HM Nano-Detox liquid by Premier Research Lab

   Key Ingredients:

- Chlorella: this type of sea algae is by far the most effective nutrient for drawing out and eliminating metals (particularly mercury). This product contains chlorella that has been broken down into very small, nano-sized particles, which greatly increases absorption and effectiveness.

Gentle Fibers by JarrowFormulas

This product assists the transport of the metals and chemical released out through the intestines.

Key Ingredients:

- Fibers/Flavonoids

- Insoluble fiber (cellulose and hemicellulose)

- Soluble fiber (pectin, mucilage)

- Flavonoids (hesperidin, naringen, limictrol)

- Lignans (from flaxseed oil)

3. Continue with these three formulas for another two weeks and then take one week off. Repeating this sequence monthly for three months is the ideal way to easily and effectively clean your body of years of accumulated environmental contaminants and toxins.

Detoxification for Infants and Children

Infants and children are still growing and developing their detoxification organs and systems. Because their liver, kidneys, intestinal system and blood-brain barrier are still under construction, they are much more susceptible to the adverse effects of pollutants and less capable of detoxifying these toxins.

There are also individual differences between children. There are children who are more susceptible to different types of toxins because their particular body may have a more difficult time detoxifying and eliminating that particular type of toxin. This is very commonly seen with metals such as lead, mercury or cadmium, where two children from the same family may have the same degree of exposure, but one child's body is unable to detoxify that metal as effectively as the other child. The first child will be the one to suffer from the effects of the exposure.

Due to these individual differences and because of the inherent sensitivity to detoxification and toxins in the childhood years, I strongly recommend that any detoxification program for your child be coordinated and overseen by a health-care professional who is particularly experienced in working with children and capable of undertaking the testing needed to design a detoxification program that is specific to your child.

Living Healthfully in a Toxic Environment

Unless you and your family are sailing peacefully around the world on your own boat, or living on a virtually uninhabited island in the middle of the Pacific Ocean, you are being exposed to the vast array of toxic chemicals and metals prevalent in today's world. The extent to which each individual and, in particular, each child, is affected by these pollutants will vary depending on overall health, nutritional status, quality of medical care, genetic predispositions and the amount of exposure.

In light of this reality, the only sensible approach is to

- Reduce your exposure to toxins whenever possible (especially in your home environment)

- Take antioxidant supplements on a regular basis to help

neutralize and detoxify the toxins that do accumulate

- Implement a cleansing and detoxifying program on a yearly basis for you, the parent, utilizing the nutrients and program listed above

These are the best ways currently available to manage toxic exposure, protecting yourself and your children, and helping to prevent the development of any adverse or serious consequences from the environment we are all living in.

"The day is near at hand when the doctor will no longer be engaged to patch up the sick man, but to prevent him from getting sick. He will visit families, examine the premises, inspect factories and shops and give instruction to his patients how to keep from getting sick".

—Boston Medical Journal 1908

Chapter 4

Choosing the Right Medical Care for Your Child

It's perfectly normal for children to catch a cold, cough or the flu occasionally. And when given the correct natural treatment, they should recover quickly, easily and completely. It is *not* normal for children to get sick frequently, catch every bug that is going around, or endure long recovery times. It is *not* normal to suffer from ongoing mucus, congestion, coughs, or recurrent ear, sinus or upper respiratory infections. And it is certainly not normal for children to require antibiotics every time they catch something.

Too often in my medical clinic, I see children who were treated by allopathic medical doctors but continue to suffer recurring ear, sinus or upper respiratory infections. Each of these infections had previously been treated with antibiotics, but within a month or two, another infection would appear. The adverse effects of antibiotic use on the immune system include impaired development of granulocytes, thrombocytes and lymphocytes, while also suppressing the action of phagocytes.[1] (*These are all immune cells, each with their own specialized function.*) Recurrent antibiotic use can cause bone marrow depression, which then impairs the development of all these important immune cells and the ability of the immune system to respond appropriately. Antibiotics are also capable of causing allergic reactions, skin eruptions and liver dysfunction.[2]

As the immune system is weakened by the repeated use of antibiotics, children become more susceptible to infection, which is then treated with another round of antibiotics—a vicious circle.

THE CORRECT MEDICAL CARE

The correct medical care and treatment is to clear the infection and other symptoms while simultaneously supporting and strengthening the immune system. With the correct medical care, your child should grow stronger after recovering from each acute infection, as his or her immune system grows "wiser" and more effective from the experience. This translates to a lower susceptibility to illness and an easier and quicker recovery without the use of antibiotics.

The purpose of this chapter is to explain the different types of medical treatment that are currently available so you will be better able to select the kind of medical care that will benefit your child the most, in the short term and the long term.

All medical conditions can be placed into one of two categories: acute or chronic. Acute conditions are short-term maladies such as colds, coughs, fevers or the flu, while chronic conditions are ongoing, longer-term problems such as recurrent ear infections, asthma, eczema, digestive problems, stomachaches, learning difficulties, behavioral and mood conditions, plus the whole spectrum of autistic disorders.

Regardless of whether your child's condition is acute or chronic, the most important issues are

- How to treat the condition

- How to help your child's immune system respond appropriately and correctly to the challenge

- How to help your child's immune system become stronger and "wiser" after each encounter

- How to help your child's immune system grow and mature properly

Ultimately, the way a condition is treated will affect how your child grows, evolves and matures into adulthood.

What Is a Symptom?

Disease and illness are typically characterized according to their symptoms. But what exactly is a symptom? Here's what Webster's Dictionary has to say:

symp-tom: (n)

1. A characteristic sign or indication of the existence of **something else.**

2. A sign or an indication of disorder or disease.

3. A phenomenon that arises from and accompanies a particular disease or disorder **and serves as an indicator of it**.

In other words, a symptom is a warning that something negative is occurring on a deeper level within the body. You can think of a symptom as the engine trouble indicator light on the dashboard of your car. When it comes on, you stop the car as soon as possible because you know that something is not functioning properly and needs to be addressed. Pretending not to see the light, or covering it up with a piece of tape, will only lead to more serious problems.

Treating the Symptom, But Not the Cause

Allopathic treatments and pharmaceutical medications do just that: they only cover up the symptom and never address the real cause of the problem. Take pneumonia, for example—an infection in the lungs. A person with pneumonia always suffers from some other condition or stressor that has weakened the immune system, made them vulnerable and allowed the pneumonia to develop. According to the American Journal of Public Health, older age and underlying disease are the most important contributing factors to developing pneumonia. Treating pneumonia with antibiotics relieves the symptoms but does nothing to address the underlying immune weakness that made the person susceptible in the first place.

Another example, commonly seen in children, is the recurrent ear infection. The typical allopathic treatment for an ear infection is a five-to-ten-day course of antibiotics. If the infection recurs a week, a month or three months later, antibiotics are given again. In cases like this, it's clear that although the medication alleviated the immediate symptom (ear infection), it didn't cure the pattern of illness because it didn't treat the real problem of the underlying immune weakness, which creates the susceptibility. And it may have made the problem even worse. Studies have shown that when ear infections are treated with antibiotics, it can lead to an actual increase in the number and frequency of ear infections.[3]

The Real Problem

The real problem with any type of recurring infection is that something is interfering with the immune system's ability to do its job. For some reason, the immune system is allowing pathogens (bacteria or viruses) to invade and is not responding appropriately. Simply suppressing the symptoms (in this case, a bacteria or virus that is growing out of control in the ear) via pharmaceutical medications may stop the immediate pain or associated fever, but it doesn't solve the root problem and often leads to the appearance of another symptom or problem. It's like squeezing a balloon in one area: the balloon just bulges in another place. When ear, sinus or upper respiratory infections are repeatedly suppressed with antibiotics, the immune system grows weaker. The problem can then travel deeper into the body, affecting more vital tissues and internal organs, and the child may then go on to develop eczema, asthma or some type of nervous disorder.[4]

Fortunately, the body will always let you know that something is wrong through the symptoms your child displays. This notification may be "diplomatic" at first, but if the warning is ignored or suppressed, the symptoms will become more obvious, distressing and uncomfortable.

Understanding the enormous difference between suppressing symptoms through pharmaceutical drugs and truly healing your child by treating the root cause is the beginning of truly effective medical care.

Don't miss the opportunity to get the correct treatment for your child. Pay attention to the message a symptom delivers.

THE HEALING MODALITIES

The balance of this chapter focuses on the various healing systems, from Western allopathic medicine to homeopathy, naturopathy, osteopathy and Oriental medicine, explaining their philosophies, treatment principles, methods, and their pros and cons. Understanding the different approaches taken by various healing professions and health practitioners can help you choose the very best medical care for your child in any situation.

Allopathic/Western Medicine

Credentials: Medical Doctor (M.D.)

"Suppress the symptom at all costs" could be the motto of the allopathic approach; the origins of the symptom are of less interest. A human being is viewed as a one-dimensional entity that can be divided into parts, which are then treated individually and separately. Typically, symptoms arising in an isolated part of the body are treated with pharmaceutical drugs prescribed by a specialist in that particular area (e.g., an allergist, gastroenterologist, dermatologist, ear, nose and throat specialist, psychiatrist and so on). The pharmaceutical drugs are usually chemically synthesized substances aimed at either stimulating or blocking a particular metabolic pathway or cellular function.

The allopathic approach has been around for at least 100 years, but the only real change seen during that time is that the drugs used to treat (suppress) the symptoms have grown stronger, more concentrated and more targeted. As a result, we see medications that have more severe side effects and the stronger suppression of symptoms eventually leads to more serious and negative long-term effects.

Allopathic medicine is at its best when utilized for treating emergency situations, such as traumatic injuries resulting from accidents or falls. It can also be an excellent choice at the other end of the spectrum, when chronic medical conditions have progressed to the point of requiring drastic measures to survive, as in cases of cancer, organ or joint failure. At times like these, surgical interventions such as heart bypasses, joint replacements, tumor removal and organ transplants can be highly effective and life-prolonging treatments. Holistic modalities and methods do not work fast enough in these drastic chronic conditions, but can be used simultaneously to assist the body in the recuperation and repair process.

Allopathic Treatment Principles and Methods:

- Develop a diagnosis by affixing a "medical-sounding" name to a particular group of symptoms

- Prescribe a pharmaceutical drug based on the name/diagnosis

- Suppress symptoms via use of this pharmaceutical drug[5]

Consequences:

- The pharmaceutical drug does not address the underlying reason for the symptoms

- The pharmaceutical drug masks the real problem or problems

- Symptom suppression eventually leads to more symptoms or increased severity of original symptoms, at the initial site or elsewhere in the body

- Additional pharmaceutical drugs are prescribed to suppress the other symptoms and conditions that arise as a consequence of the initial treatment

Pros:

- Best treatment for traumatic injuries (e.g., broken bones, lacerations)

- Also good for end-stage, life-threatening conditions such as organ failure, and surgical interventions for cancer, or for alleviation of long-term wear and tear conditions such as joint damage and replacement

Cons:

- The condition or disorder is never treated properly except in the case of acute injuries and broken bones.

- There is usually increased toxicity, distress and disorder due to side effects of the treatment, including severe drug side effects.

- Apart from the cases of acute injury, trauma and broken bones, the individual never gets completely well because the underlying causal issues that need to be addressed are ignored.

- It is completely focused on disease and never on health.

Successful Treatment

James was only 2 years old and already he had a long history of recurrent infections. He had been treated with antibiotics repeatedly over the past year for recurrent upper respiratory infections and bacterial infections on his skin.

The upper respiratory infections had continued to reoccur despite the antibiotics and were now developing into asthma-like symptoms, which required breathing treatments and a steroid inhaler in addition to the antibiotics.

James's immune system was declining rapidly with the continual cycles of antibiotics and consequently, his symptoms were going deeper by moving from upper respiratory infections into asthma. This is exactly what happens when the symptoms are suppressed: the immune system is weakened further and the problem travels deeper into the body.

After looking at his medical history, personality and the characteristics of his own particular nature, he was prescribed his homeopathic constitutional remedy, Calcarea Carbonica 9 c, to be taken once daily, and the nutritional supplements of colostrum, probiotics, vitamin C and vitamin D3 to start repairing and strengthening his immune system.

At his six-week follow up visit, his mother reported that he had started catching a cold one month after starting the remedy and treatment, but for the first time in a year it did not progress into an infection, and he didn't require any breathing treatments. By increasing the dosage of his remedy and supplements for a few days, he was able to fight off the cold symptoms and return to normal.

James continues taking his homeopathic remedy and nutritional supplements, and I would expect it will take about a year of this treatment for his immune system to fully recover and be back to full strength.

Holistic Medicine

"Holistic medicine" is often used as a catchall term for any alternative system of medicine. In reality, it refers to certain approaches to medicine rather than a specific system—specifically, approaches that view the individual as a whole, rather than a sum of individual physical organs, and emphasizes the connection between body, mind and spirit. Homeopathic medicine, nutritional medicine, naturopathic medicine and osteopathic medicine are just a few of the disciplines that belong within the larger category of holistic medicine.

Homeopathic Medicine

*Credentials: Master Homeopath (M.Hom.), Certified Classical
Homeopath (CCH), or Registered Society of Homeopathy (RSHom)*

Homeopathy is a medical method, science and art that centers on a
comprehensive view of the individual, which allows treatment and
healing on the deepest possible physical, emotional and spiritual
levels. It is based on the principle of "like cures like," which has
a documented history of application dating back to Hippocrates,
and even 2,500 years ago to Moses and the Old Testament. The
substance that creates the symptoms of a specific illness in a
healthy person is used in a very diluted form to heal that disease
in a sick person; thus, "like cures like."

In 1810, Samuel Hahnemann, M.D., became the first "modern"
physician to apply this principle and develop a scientific method
of selecting and prescribing the one single correct "remedy" for
each individual case. He did this by conducting clinical trials
that he called "provings": giving a particular substance to
healthy people with no symptoms and observing any effects that
occurred. By noting in detail the effects of each substance on
the physical, emotional, and mental characteristics of various
healthy individuals, he started compiling a precise portfolio for the
prescribing indications of each of these substances, which he then
called "remedies."

Hahnemann also detailed the precise method for making these
remedies, which involves a series of steps for diluting the original
substance to be able to gain all the good effects while avoiding any
toxic side effects. Each particular "remedy" is made into a liquid
dilution that is then placed onto and absorbed into small white
pellets, which are then taken by dissolving under the tongue.
The homeopathic medicine chest now contains these precise
portraits and indications for over 2,000 remedies or substances.

The methods and principles of homeopathic medicine were meticulously detailed in Hahnemann's treatise, *The Organon of Medicine*, which was first published in 1810 and continues to be published today. Healing on the deepest physical, emotional and spiritual level can occur when homeopathic medicine is applied and prescribed correctly according to Hahnemann's methods and principles.

The homeopath's job is to select and prescribe one precise remedy for an individual's illness based on that person's physical, emotional, and mental characteristics. The homeopath should also take into account the spiritual patterns that are reflected in that individual's life. The one single correct remedy prescribed by the homeopath is called a "constitutional" remedy. It has the potential, over time, to treat all aspects of the individual and heal the deeper emotional and spiritual disturbances that usually lie at the origin of physical symptoms and disorders.

There is a great deal of variation in the way that homeopathic medicine is utilized by doctors and practitioners. Some use the remedies in a superficial way, aiming them at symptom relief much as a medical doctor would use a pharmaceutical drug. This is *not* the way homeopathic treatments were intended to be applied. It is important to find a homeopath who is trained in "Hahnemannian Homeopathy" and prescribes homeopathic remedies from a constitutional perspective.

Homeopathic Treatment Principles and Methods:

- Observe and evaluate all physical, emotional, mental and spiritual characteristics and patterns of the patient.

- Based on this evaluation, select and prescribe one of the 2,000 homeopathic remedies. This one single ("constitutional") remedy is the substance that best matches all of the individual's characteristics.

- The "constitutional" remedy is taken daily or periodically at a specific dosage and potency that is adjusted as healing occurs.

- Homeopathic remedies can also be given for acute situations such as a cold, cough, sore throat, food poisoning, after an injury or after surgery to assist healing.

Consequences:

- Healing in the most thorough and natural way without any unwanted side effects.

Pros:

- Potential for complete healing in the deepest possible way, with long-lasting benefits

- Healing of current conditions and maintenance of true health and vitality

- Over time, a change in the actions or attitudes that may have been contributing to discord and disease

Cons:

- The full benefits of "constitutional" homeopathy occur over time; it is a process that takes understanding and patience.

- The correct "constitutional" remedy needs to be prescribed by a well-educated and experienced homeopath. Unfortunately, there are too few of these.

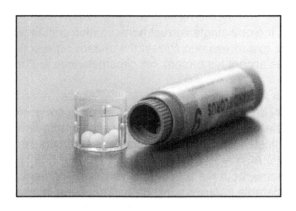

Successful Treatment

Charles was 7 years old when his mother first brought him to see me at my clinic.

Overall, he had been in good health, catching the occasional cold andfever, and one previous ear infection.

His parents were health conscious, providing a healthy diet with very little fast foods and sugars.

Charles's difficulties began to occur after his younger brother was born. At first, it was just some over-attentive and forceful holding and hugs towards his newborn brother. However, this soon developed into more aggressive behavior: he began hitting and striking his brother when he thought he could get away with it. This behavior soon began to show up at school, as well, with Charles getting into conflicts and fights and always being the first one to lash out and physically hit the other children. Around this same time, Charles also showed some difficulties with focusing and learning at school.

The concerned teachers and school principal talked to Charles's parents about his behavior and learning difficulties and as a result, I saw him in my clinic.

Looking at his previous health history and the family's healthy habits and lifestyle, this appeared to be purely an emotional issue, whereby his jealousy and frustration about his younger brother were pushing his slight mean streak into a bigger mean streak and manifesting into conflicts, fighting and hitting. This type of emotional distress can also affect the nervous system and therefore interfere with focus and learning.

In this situation, the one single correct homeopathic constitutional remedy worked wonders to address and correct the underlying emotional conflicts and help Charles accept his brother, his circumstances and move on in life.

For this behavior I prescribed the homeopathic remedy nitric acid 6c to be given once a day on a daily basis, with a follow up in six weeks' time. After the six weeks, the parents had noticed some slight improvements with less hitting, so we adjusted the dosage and continued with the same remedy.

Within three months, both the school teachers and Charles's parents had observed considerable improvement. He had not been involved in any fights at school, even when provoked. He had stopped hitting his younger brother and after another two months, he was catching up with the reading and math skills that he had previously fallen behind on.

A straightforward case for a homeopathic constitutional remedy.

Nutritional Medicine

Credentials: Nutritional medicine (also known as orthomolecular medicine) is usually practiced by naturopathic, medical, chiropractic or osteopathic physicians who have received additional and specialized training in orthomolecular medicine.

During the 20th century, new scientific methods made it possible to observe the inner workings of the human body more closely. We began to learn a lot more about nutrients—the building blocks of both body and brain, and the substances that are necessary for proper body functions. This research and knowledge gave birth to the relatively new science of nutritional medicine.

Linus Pauling, Ph.D, a two-time Nobel laureate, is considered by many to be the father of this field[6], and was the first to map the internal pathways of many nutrient functions and utilization. The original advocate of the health benefits of vitamin C, Pauling recommended taking large daily doses of vitamin C, for which he was heavily criticized by the allopathic medical community. Linus

Pauling easily outlived all of his critics and detractors, taking large doses of vitamin C on a daily basis and living with full function and vitality to the age of 96.

Another founder of nutritional medicine is Weston Price, D.D.S, a dentist and outstanding medical researcher who was the first to study the negative impact of modern processed foods on the human body. By observing many native peoples in different countries and cultures at the beginning of the 1900s, he documented the rapid decline in health that began to occur when these native cultures started replacing their traditional foods and diet with processed sugars, processed grains and processed fats. Price's photographic documentation, which appears in his book *Nutrition and Physical Degeneration* (1939), shows the dramatic and harmful impact that these dietary changes created in the facial features, bones, teeth, physique and overall health of these cultures and populations in the relatively short time span of one generation.

To apply nutritional medicine, the physician assesses both body and brain from a holistic perspective, determining which tissues, glands or organs are associated with the presenting symptoms or complaints. Through tests and evaluation of the various functions of the affected tissues, the physician can decide which vitamins, minerals, fatty acids, amino acids and enzymes will help these tissues and organs detoxify, rejuvenate and return to proper function.

Treatment Principles and Methods:

- Evaluate the nutritional status of the individual through urine, blood, stool and hair analysis.

- Determine if any imbalances, deficiencies or toxicities exist.

- Provide specific nutrients (vitamins, minerals, essential fatty acids, amino acids, probiotics, enzymes and co-factors) based on the individual's symptoms and associated test results.

- These nutrients can target and strengthen tissues, organs, or pathways wherever the help is required.

- Proactively supplement with antioxidants and other nutrients that protect the body against toxins and pollutants.

- Give only those nutrients that already exist in the body, to decrease the risk of toxicity or side effects associated with pharmaceutical or herbal medicines.

Consequences:

- The body's own natural healing mechanisms have an opportunity to correct any underlying problems when given the correct support.

- The body is detoxified and protected against the effects of environmental pollution and toxicity.

- The body and brain receive the optimum amount of essential nutrients.

- Health improvement, maintenance and prevention.

Pros:

- There are usually never any side effects because only nutrients that already exist in the body are given.

- The optimal amount of nutrients allows the internal organs and cells to function at their full potential.

- It is a great way to optimize health, providing nutrients for optimal growth, development, maturation and longevity.

Cons:

- Does not address any underlying emotional, mental or spiritual discord that may be contributing to the symptoms.

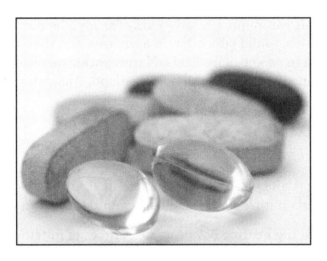

Naturopathic Medicine

Credentials: Naturopathic Doctor (N.D.)

Naturopathic medicine has its roots in the fields of diet, nutrition, exercise and herbal medicine. The term "naturopathy" was first used by an American, John Scheel, in the 1890s, and the first official naturopathic medical school was opened in New York in 1905. Many of those in North America and abroad who became naturopathic doctors were medical doctors dismayed by the methods, toxic medicines and harmful results that traditional allopathic medical practices had inflicted on patients. Interested in finding safer alternatives and more natural methods, they discovered that correcting the diet, engaging in daily exercise, making certain lifestyle changes and using therapeutic hydrotherapy (hot and cold baths and mineral springs) could lead to a marked improvement in an individual's health. Naturopathic doctors also utilized herbal botanical medicines, emphasizing the prescription of herbs that grew locally.

Today's naturopathic doctor is trained in nutrition, diet, exercise, methods of physical manipulation, botanical/herbal medicine, homeopathy, as well as the basics of allopathic medicine. As each of these fields can require many years of study, the naturopathic doctor receives a solid education in each area and then may go on to specialize in one or more fields. Naturopathic medical schools are now found in America, Canada, England, Australia and New Zealand.

Treatment Principles and Methods:

- Support and encourage the innate healing powers of the body via nature's own medicines and methods.

- Utilize the healing power and resources of nutrition and nature

- Evaluate nutritional status, diet and food choices.

- Test for toxic buildup of metals, chemicals and other industrial pollutants within the body.

- Assess function and ecology of the digestive system and intestinal integrity.

- Screen for emotional, mental or situational stresses that may be contributing to illness.

Consequences:

- Allows the body to recover naturally in its own way and at its own rate.

- Establishes healthy dietary and exercise habits that can provide a foundation for good health over a lifetime.

- Emphasizes maintenance of health and prevention of illness (which should be the focus of every path of medicine).

Pros:

- Natural healing leads to a stronger body, mind and spirit.

- Healthy habits and patterns create and sustain health over a lifetime.

- An N.D. is a well-rounded physician with education, training, experience and expertise in a wide range of modalities. He or she can be a great physician and a great ally for your child's health.

Cons:

- None. If the N.D. is able to prescribe the correct homeopathic "constitutional" remedy, in addition to utilizing the other modalities of diet, nutrition and supplementation, then you have a physician with a very broad and great set of skills and knowledge with no deficiency or downside.

Osteopathic Medicine

Credentials: Doctor of Osteopathy (D.O.)

Osteopathy was developed in 1874 by the American medical doctor Andrew Taylor Still. Dismayed at the poor results and serious harm often caused by traditional medical practices, Dr. Still sought a deeper understanding of what caused illness and how to heal more completely. Through his studies, he discovered that the body healed most efficiently when its blood, lymphatic, cerebrospinal fluid, and nerve and energy pathways were cleared of obstructions. When all of these systems were free to distribute messages, immune factors, energy and nutrients, the body was then able to heal and remain healthy and strong. Thus, keeping all of the body's systems free of obstructions appeared to be the key to good health.

To facilitate the clearing of such obstructions, Dr. Still developed a sophisticated system of hands-on physical manipulation techniques known as osteopathic manipulative treatment (OMT). The exact spot where an obstruction lies must be discovered, and then the osteopath uses OMT to unblock and release it.

In America, a Doctor of Osteopathy (D.O.) receives the equivalent education and prescribing privileges as a Medical Doctor, (M.D.) with the added benefit of additional training and skills in Osteopathic Manipulative Techniques.

Osteopathic Manipulative Treatments

There are four basic kinds of OMT:

1. *Soft tissue manipulation* – Used to evaluate the condition of the connective tissue and help the body's blood and lymphatic fluids flow smoothly.

2. *Osteopathic articular technique* – Used to reduce muscle spasms or nerve irritation affecting a joint, to make joints more mobile and reduce any associated pain and discomfort.

3. *Cranial osteopathy* – Used to assess and treat the mobility of the skull and ensure smooth and unrestricted flow of the cerebrospinal fluid, thereby synchronizing and stabilizing the body's innate biorhythms.

4. *Visceral manipulation* – Used to treat the internal organs of the body, improve the mobility of an organ, increase blood

flow and nerve conduction, and help the organs function more effectively.

With an excellent education in anatomy, physiology and all associated systems in the body, plus a great deal of practice, the osteopath develops a finely honed ability to determine the location of any congestion, restriction or obstruction in the body. In fact, a skilled osteopath may be able to lay his or her hands on an adult patient and determine that the patient fell off his bike at the age of 6, landed on his left shoulder, then struck the left side of his head and is still affected today by the compaction and distortion from this accident.

Osteopaths specialize in adjusting and manipulating both body and brain to correct imbalances, poor alignment or obstructions that interfere with the normal flow of fluids and nourishment throughout your nervous system, immune system and body. In the case of children, all babies should see an osteopathic doctor within their first month or two after birth to determine whether anything is out of alignment and, if so, gently realign and correct it. Just imagine the trauma inflicted on a child's head during the birth process. The infant's skull is not one piece of bone, but rather four separate pieces that fit together via expansion and contraction joints. Depending on your child's position and the time spent in the birth canal, different forces and pressures will be exerted on these delicate cranial plates. This can create compaction and compression resulting in misalignment, which can affect how well the brain will grow and function. Any unresolved compaction may contribute to recurrent ear infections, sleep disorders, difficulty walking, delayed development, problems with focus and learning, mood disorders and many other conditions.[7]

But there need not be any symptoms present to warrant an osteopathic treatment for your child. Remember: the best medicine is preventative, and it is an excellent idea to see an osteopath for maintenance and prevention, to remove any obstructions and keep all systems flowing *before* they have a chance to create a problem.

Treatment Principles and Methods:

- Determine the exact location of any congestion or obstruction in the blood, lymphatic, cerebrospinal fluid, nerve and energy pathways.

- Gently remove these obstructions through the use of specific, hands-on osteopathic manipulative techniques.

Consequences:

- When the blood, lymphatic and cerebrospinal fluids, nerve and energy pathways are unobstructed, the body is able to rejuvenate and regenerate where needed to maintain an active, vital state of health.

- When combined with well-prescribed homeopathy and nutritional supplementation, osteopathy offers the finest and the highest level of natural medicine and natural healing methods.

Pros:

- The body has the opportunity to tap into its own innate healing abilities.

- Potential problems can be corrected before they become real trouble or create obvious symptoms.

Cons:

- Does not address spiritual discord that may be present.

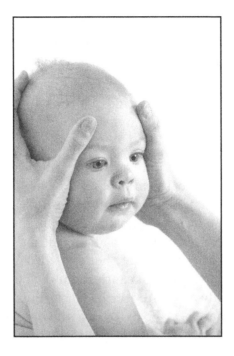

Infant receiving ostepathic treatment

Herbal Medicine

Credentials: Herbal medicine, also known as botanical medicine, may be prescribed by a Naturopathic Doctor (N.D.) Licensed Acupuncturist (L.Ac.), or Master Herbalist (M.H.).

Every country and culture in the world has a tradition of using local plants or plant parts (collectively referred to as herbs) for medicinal purposes. These plants typically are not part of the everyday diet because they contain chemical substances that would be harmful if eaten continually or in large amounts. When taken in the proper amounts, however, these chemical substances can affect the body in beneficial ways. For example, St. John's

Wort is known to improve mood and fight viral infections. Olive leaf extract contains oleic acid, which has strong antibacterial, antiviral and antifungal properties. Milk thistle (silymarin) has strong detoxifying and cleansing effects on the liver. Echinacea stimulates the immune system by increasing the activity of various kinds of immune cells. Vinpocetine, which is extracted from the periwinkle plant, assists and improves memory.

When the pharmaceutical industry began in the early 1900s, the majority of pharmaceutical drugs were based on compounds extracted from herbs, which were then synthetically reproduced in the laboratory under trademark protection. Thus, herbal medicine is more closely related to allopathic medicine and its pharmaceutical drugs than other "holistic" disciplines. Because they can act much like pharmaceuticals in the body, herbal medicines should always be prescribed or formulated by a medical practitioner who has received extensive and specialized training in this field. It is also crucial that herbal medicines be taken at the prescribed dosage and for the recommended amount of time only.

Three Kinds of Herbal Medicine

There are three major herbal traditions, each with its own medical system of application and history:

Chinese herbal medicine dates back over 4,000 years to 2,500 B.C. and includes a pharmacy of around 350 individual herbs. Herbal formulas and methods for diagnosing and applying these herbs have been taught and applied in Asia for thousands of years. The Chinese herbalist prescribes a formula based on the presenting symptoms, evaluating the characteristics of all six pulses that exist in Chinese medicine and observation of the tongue. The formula will often be a combination of several different herbs designed to work together to address the symptoms by targeting the organs and tissues involved in the condition.[8]

Ayurvedic medicine originated in India and dates back to around 1000 B.C. The ayurvedic practitioner uses a specific method of evaluation and diagnosis, and then prescribes the appropriate herbal formula. A number of traditional ayurvedic formulas have long been used to treat specific conditions, or the practitioner may create a formula customized to the individual person and problem, choosing from some 500 herbs and substances.

Western herbal medicine is a medicinal system created in the Western world (Europe, North America and South America) utilizing the plants and herbs that grow in these areas. The first known author of a classification system for plants in Europe was Theophrastus, who lived around 300 B.C. Dioscorides (40-90 A.D.) compiled the first book of medicinal herbal medicine in his *Materia Medica*, which became the primary reference for later herbal medicine textbooks, beginning in the 16th century. Historically, use of these herbs and formulas was based on the experience of the practitioner through application, observation and results. Over the past 30 years, many of these herbs have now been studied in the laboratory and the active ingredients and compounds have been isolated and understood. In addition to the whole plants and herbs prescribed in formulas, today's herbalist may also recommend individual herbs or standardized extracts for specific conditions.

Treatment Principles and Methods:

- **Chinese herbalists** diagnose the underlying condition based on symptoms and observation of the tongue, pulse, and physical and emotional characteristics, and then prescribe an herbal formula that may contain several herbs.

- **Ayurvedic herbalists** diagnose the underlying condition based on the symptoms, body measurements, diet suitability, digestive capacity, physical fitness, features and age, and then prescribe an herbal formula based on these characteristics.

- **Western herbalists** diagnose the underlying illness based on the presenting physical symptoms and history, and then prescribe an herbal formula that may contain several herbs.

Consequences:

- Herbs exert healing, stimulating, soothing or other effects on target tissues and organs.

- If prescribed correctly, they will have a beneficial effect on the condition, at least during the treatment period, with minimum side effects.

Pros:

- A correctly prescribed herbal formula will exert corrective action relatively quickly.

- Less toxicity than pharmaceutical drugs when prescribed correctly.

Cons:

- Herbal extracts can vary in strength and concentration depending on when and where they were grown and harvested.

- There may be side effects, as herbal medicines are similar to pharmaceutical drugs.

- Continued or prolonged use of an herb or herbal formula may create symptoms or increase the very symptoms you are trying to correct.

- Herbal medicine does not address the underlying emotional or spiritual discord that may be contributing to the symptoms.

Note: *Long-term use of herbal formulas should always be overseen by a well-educated and experienced health-care professional who specializes in herbal medicine.*

For acute conditions like a cough, cold or the flu, herbal remedies can be used very safely and effectively for brief periods of time (i.e., 10 to 14 days). Chronic conditions such as eczema or dermatitis, digestive problems, reflux, colic, constipation, immune disorders, allergies, recurrent infections, behavioral disorders or conditions related to the autistic spectrum are best treated with homeopathic remedies in combination with dietary adjustments and nutritional supplementation.

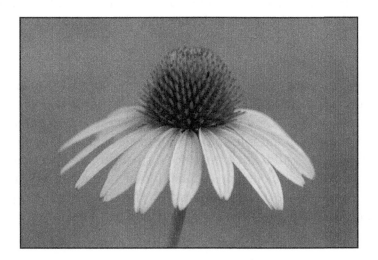

Chiropractic

Credentials: Doctor of Chiropractic (D.C.)

Chiropractic medicine, like osteopathic medicine, involves physical adjustment of the body. A major difference between the two is that chiropractic adjustments are focused primarily on the spine, rather than the whole body.

Created in 1895 as an independent form of medicine by Daniel Palmer, an American healer, chiropractic is now a well-established form of medical treatment in many countries. It is based on the idea that the spine, the primary conduit of the nervous system, must be kept properly aligned and free of obstructions (subluxations) in order to work properly. Daniel Palmer "discovered" chiropractic while treating a janitor who worked in his office building. The janitor told Palmer that 17 years earlier he had felt something "give" in his back when he bent over, and almost immediately he began losing his hearing. Upon examining his back, Palmer found a protruding vertebra in his upper spine. When Palmer pushed the vertebra back into position, the janitor suddenly began to hear more clearly. The first chiropractic adjustment had just occurred![9]

But spinal manipulation is nothing new. The earliest written account dates back to 2700 B.C., found in a Chinese document called the Kou Fou. Later, the Greek physicians Hippocrates and Galen practiced spinal manipulation and recognized its importance in relation to overall health. In 19th century Europe and America, the "bonesetters" (physicians and healers who specialized in physical and structural manipulations) played a prominent part in health care. Chiropractic is an extension of all of the above.

Treatment Principles and Methods:

- Use physical adjustments to remove any congestion or obstructions (subluxations) in the spine that may be affecting the flow of information and energy throughout the central nervous system.

Consequences:

- Removing spinal obstructions releases the body's own healing energy, which can be applied to any ongoing conditions or symptoms.

- The individual can participate in self-healing by experiencing the changes that take place after the adjustment.

Pros:

- If the symptoms are related to or associated with subluxations in the spinal column, chiropractic adjustment can exert broad and profound benefits.

- Chiropractic contributes to health maintenance and the prevention of disease by keeping everything in the body in good working order.

Cons:

- The effects may not be as all-encompassing or profound as those seen in some osteopathic treatments.

- Chiropractic may not address any spiritual discord that may be contributing to the condition.

Children in need of spinal realignment or adjustment generally require a gentle and specialized treatment. When seeking chiropractic care for your child, it is important to find a practitioner who specializes in treating children and who works extensively with them.

Acupuncture

Credentials: Licensed Acupuncturist (L.Ac.), Doctor of Acupuncture (D.Ac.)

Acupuncture, the insertion of very thin needles into specific anatomical points on the body, dates back to 2000 B.C. and is perhaps the oldest, most well-documented system of medicine in the world. It is based on the precept that energy is the most important component of the body. Energy regulates all of the functions and processes in the body. Nothing occurs without the presence of energy, just as a match doesn't light until the energy of movement strikes it against a flint.

The circulation of energy throughout the body occurs via special pathways called meridians, which affect and regulate every organ in our bodies. The points at which these meridians come closest to the surface of the skin are the acupuncture points, each of which affects specific bodily functions.[10]

Based on a comprehensive evaluation of symptoms, pulse, tongue, and physical and emotional characteristics, the acupuncturist ascertains which acupuncture points must be stimulated to accomplish the desired effects.

Treatment Principles and Methods:

- Determine acupuncture points that need stimulation to unblock meridians and allow energy to circulate.

- Insert acupuncture needles into these points to remove blockages and increase movement of energy to specific vessels, tissues, organs or glands.

Consequences:

- Unblocking of energy allows the body's own healing mechanisms and vital force to address and correct the underlying causes of symptoms.

- The body's innate healing abilities are stimulated.

- Complete healing can occur when acupuncture is given correctly.

Pros:

- Both body and spirit (which exists in energy form) can be treated

- Offers pure energetic healing

- Effective for acute and chronic conditions, as well as health maintenance and disease prevention

Cons:

- Not all acupuncturists are trained to treat the deepest part of the individual's being—the spirit/soul.

- In today's world, nutritional supplementation and detoxification is usually required along with acupuncture to affect complete healing.

I have a particular fondness and appreciation for acupuncture, which was the first discipline I learned in my medical training. However, I have found that for children, homeopathy and homeopathic remedies are a much more practical approach. It is a lot easier and more effective to give a baby or child homeopathic pellets or drops that easily dissolve in the mouth than it is to insert and maintain the position of acupuncture needles, which require a period of stillness.

Note: Since acupuncture and homeopathy both work on a deep level through the energy system, you need not use both methods at once. Choose one and stay with it to see the results.

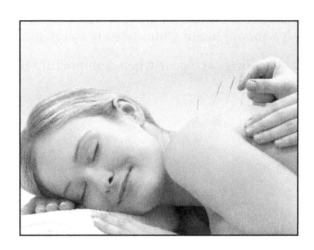

Dentistry (Bio-Compatible)

Credentials: Doctor of Dental Surgery (D.D.S.), Doctor of Dental Medicine, (D.M.D.)

The mouth is intricately connected to the body and situated close to the brain. It follows that everything that goes into the mouth or the teeth will impact the rest of the body, including the brain. Yet it is amazing how many dentists overlook or simply disregard this connection when they fill dental cavities with mercury and other toxic materials. In dentistry, these fillings are misleadingly called "dental amalgams," although they should be called "mercury amalgams," as mercury makes up 50 percent of their content, in addition to silver, tin, copper and zinc.[11]

All of these metals are potentially neurotoxic, meaning they can damage and kill brain cells[12], but mercury is the most worrisome.

It is one of the most toxic metals on earth, comparable in toxicity to lead or arsenic. When mercury is used in a work environment or involved in the manufacture of any product, it is always classified as a highly toxic, highly poisonous substance, and there are strict rules and regulations as to how it can be transported, handled and disposed.[13] Yet, somehow, all of this dangerous and harmful toxicity continues to be ignored by many in the dental profession and mercury continues to be placed in the teeth of millions of Americans, even though study after study has shown that it will leak into the body.[14]

In addition, these metals can also create a galvanic (electric) current when they come in contact with the saliva, essentially creating a small battery in the mouth. These galvanic currents can be measured in microvolts and are sometimes high enough to interfere with the immune system, nervous system and brain function.[15] These potential problems can be completely eliminated by requesting that your family dentist never use any type of metal in your child's mouth and always use white composite material when filling your child's teeth.

The Truth About Mercury

The scientific literature clearly shows that

- Mercury is a highly toxic substance, whether outside or inside the mouth.

- Mercury is particularly toxic to brain cells and kidneys.

- Mercury is released and continues to be released from amalgam fillings through chewing, salivation and vaporization inside the mouth.[16]

- Some people are able to detoxify and excrete mercury better than others and are therefore less likely to have associated ill-effects.

- Those whose bodies do not detoxify and excrete mercury well, or who are very sensitive to it, are more likely to suffer adverse effects and the severe symptoms of mercury poisoning.

In April 2008, Norway, Sweden and Denmark completely banned the use of mercury in dentistry. Erik Solheim, the Norwegian minister of the environment, said that the reason for the ban is the risk that mercury poses to people and the environment. He continued, "...Mercury is among the most dangerous environmental toxins. Satisfactory alternatives to mercury in products are now available, and it is therefore fitting to introduce a ban."[17]

Germany and Austria have introduced restrictions on the use of mercury amalgams, specifically prohibiting their use in children and pregnant women. Although it seems incomprehensible, the dental communities in most other countries, including the United States, continue to insist that mercury is completely safe and carries no associated health risks.

Concerned dentists from many countries around the world have created the International Academy of Oral Medicine and Toxicology (IAOMT), an organization for dental professionals who are interested in the intimate and important relationship between the teeth, mouth and the rest of the body. The IAOMT advocates the use of blood tests to determine the biological compatibility of the many dental materials that are now available. These tests can precisely identify what particular dental products are most compatible and safe for each individual child or adult, before any material is placed into your child's mouth. If your child needs cavities filled, orthodontics, a crown or a root canal, find a dentist who recognizes the dangers of mercury and utilizes these tests to advise you regarding the safest and most biocompatible dental materials. The original blood test for biological compatibility of dental materials was developed by Clifford Research Lab, based in Colorado, U.S.A., and is now known as Clifford Materials Reactivity Testing (CMRT).[18]

Dental care is an extremely important part of your child's medical care. Making the right choices along the way can help you avoid the health problems associated with placing toxic dental materials directly into your child's mouth.

LEARN ALL YOU CAN

Providing excellent medical care is a crucial part of building a solid foundation for good health, and can be one of the greatest gifts you can give your child. Understanding the ways in which these medical disciplines approach health treatment and maintenance will help you make a more informed decision about the best kind of medical care for your child in any given situation. The golden rule is; never suppress a symptom.

Healing is a matter of time, but it is also a matter of opportunity.
—Hippocrates

Chapter 5

Vaccinations: Facts, Fears and Fallacies

The only wholly safe vaccine is the vaccine that is never used.
—Dr. J. Shannon, National Institutes of Health,
June 23, 1955

WHAT IS A VACCINATION?

A vaccination is a method of purposely introducing a foreign antigen ("germ") into the body to provoke an immune response. This response includes the production of specific antibodies to that "germ" so that the body will be able to recognize and marshal a defense against it more easily in the future.

The first documented instance of people inoculating themselves with mild doses of infectious substances to prevent a more serious infection dates back to around 200 B.C. in China.[1] In the 18th century Western world, doctors began trying to prevent smallpox by taking fluid from the pustules of a person with the disease and inserting it into a cut in the skin of a healthy person. At best, the person came down with a mild case of smallpox that conferred lifelong immunity. At worst, he or she developed a full-blown smallpox infection.

In 1796, Edward Jenner began inoculating people with cowpox fluid (taken from cows) rather than smallpox fluid (taken from humans), because he had noticed that cow maids, who had contracted the less serious disease cowpox, seemed to be immune to the potentially fatal smallpox. This approach made vaccinations somewhat safer: if they failed, the patient would contract the less dangerous disease. Another one hundred years passed before the first attempt was made to vaccinate people with a weakened culture of the virus, rather than fluid containing the "full-strength" virus.

Today, worldwide vaccination campaigns have greatly reduced the incidence of certain infectious diseases such as pertussis and diptheria, and virtually eradicated a few others, including smallpox and polio, at least for the time being. However, these same vaccines have also contributed to the well-documented and frightening increase in the incidence of childhood chronic diseases, directly causing childhood diabetes[2], autism[3], learning disorders[4], rheumatoid arthritis[5], allergies[6] and immune deficiencies[7]. In spite of this documentation, all parents are routinely urged and many times bullied by their allopathic physicians to vaccinate their newborns, and continue vaccinating their children throughout their early years.

The "Germ Theory" of Disease

In 1877, a French microbiologist named Louis Pasteur proposed the "germ theory" of disease. This theory generated the myth that all disease is caused by either a viral or bacterial infection—in other words, by a germ.[8] The doctor's job, then, was to identify the germ and kill it, which would make the disease vanish. This is a tidy theory, but it assumes that there is a neat, one-to-one correspondence between disease and germs, which is not the case.

At about the same time in history, another French microbiologist named Antoine Bechamp proposed the theory that susceptibility to disease is less a matter of exposure to germs than *it is a failure in the immune system to fight off those germs.*[9] Whether or not the body succumbs to disease depends on how clean, strong and ecologically balanced it is, how well it functions and how capable the whole immune system is able to respond to any and all challenges that come along.

Antibiotics and vaccinations are the methods that Western allopathic medicine has developed and continues to utilize in following the "germ theory" of disease. Antibiotics do kill the bacteria and vaccinations against the viruses. However, time and the ever-increasing number of children and adults suffering from chronic ongoing medical conditions continues to prove that Bechamp was correct when he said that it is the overall state, health and function of the whole body and whole immune system that is most important in determining the degree of health or sickness that we will experience over the course of a lifetime, as opposed to the ability to target a few specific bacteria and create protection from a handful of viruses with vaccinations.

Allopathic medicine continues to focus on killing the germ, not enhancing the body's own immune system.

With the advent of antibiotics in the 1940s, allopathic doctors were able to knock out many bacterial infections. But because antibiotics are completely ineffective against viruses, they have no way of addressing many viral infections. Instead, medical science has pursued and developed more and more vaccines to "prevent" the most common viral infections. Today, infants in the U.S. and many other parts of the Western world (including New Zealand) routinely receive 32 doses of 12 to 14 different vaccines before the age of 2. By age 6, this figure increases to 48 doses of 14 vaccines. Yet only 50 years earlier, a total of only 5 doses were given.

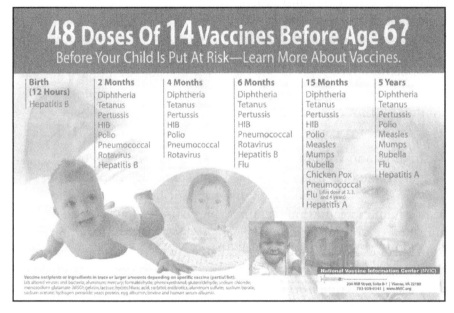

Online at http://www.nvic.org

Vaccines – A Timeline

1896 - Cholera and typhoid vaccines developed

1914 - Rabies and typhoid vaccines licensed in U.S.

1915 - Pertussis vaccine developed

1927 - BCG vaccine for tuberculosis used in newborns

1942 - Influenza A/B vaccine introduced

1943 - Penicillin mass-produced

1949 - Diptheria, tetanus and pertussis (DTP) vaccine licensed

1955 - Polio vaccine introduced

1961 - Oral polio vaccines developed

1965 - Measles vaccine introduced and licensed

1967 - Mumps vaccine introduced

1971 - Combined measles, mumps and rubella (MMR) introduced

1977 - Pneumococcal vaccine licensed

1981 - Hepatitis B viral vaccines introduced

1985 - Haemophilus influenzae type b (Hib) introduced

1995 - Varicella (chickenpox) virus vaccine introduced

1995 - Hepatitis A viral vaccine introduced

1998 - Rotavirus vaccine licensed for use in infants

2002 - Vaccine combining diptheria, tetanus, acellular pertussis, inactivated polio and hepatitis B introduced

2005 - Vaccine combining measles, mumps, rubella, and varicella (chickenpox) introduced[10]

2007 - Average number of vaccines routinely given to U.S. infants and children reaches 32 doses of 12 to 14 vaccines before 2 years of age, increasing to 48 doses of 14 vaccines by the age of 6 years[11]

AN INSIDE LOOK AT VACCINES

At first glance it's an enticing idea: inoculate children in early childhood so their immune systems will create antibodies to specific viruses (as well as certain bacteria), and these children won't contract these diseases. Yet important questions remain:

- What risks do these vaccinations pose?

- How many vaccinations can each child safely handle?

- What are the complications that can occur with each vaccine?

- Which children are more likely to suffer from adverse reactions?

- Have any of these vaccines been tested individually and collectively for long-term safety and consequences?

- Do vaccinations provide immunity to a few select infections but weaken the overall integrity of the immune system?

Each one of the above questions will be answered within this chapter. Once you've familiarized yourself with this information, you will be in a much better situation to make your own, well-informed choices.

A detailed discussion of each of the most common vaccines currently in use, plus a risk assessment, can be found in Appendix II: Rating the Vaccines.

To give you a better understand of vaccines in general, the following is a discussion of the manufacturing, ingredients and additives of vaccines.

Turning a Virus or Bacteria into a Vaccine

All vaccines begin as a virus or bacteria that is grown or cultured.

Viruses and bacteria are living organisms and they can only grow and reproduce on living tissues. The most commonly used tissues for culturing the viruses and bacteria used in vaccines are chicken embryos, aborted human fetal tissue, sheep's blood, monkey's kidneys, cow serum and monkey fetal lung cells.[12]

After the virus or bacteria has grown and matured to a certain point, it is taken from the culture and weakened in one of the following ways:

1. *Modified* – The virus or bacteria is genetically modified so that it does not reproduce so quickly.

2. *Inactivated* – The virus or bacteria is deactivated or killed with a chemical, rendering it unable to cause the disease but still able to be identified by the immune system to provoke an immunological response by the body.

3. *Cut up* - The portion of the virus or bacteria that provokes an immune response is isolated and used in the vaccine. (Hepatitis B vaccine is made this way.) For other vaccines, such as the Haemophilus influenzae B (Hib), part of the bacteria's outer membrane or wall is used.[12]

4. *Bacterial toxin* – The symptoms of inflammation and infection that are triggered by a bacterial infection are usually caused by the waste products or toxins that the bacterium releases into the body. For that reason, some bacterial vaccines are made from the bacteria's excreted toxin, which is deactivated with a chemical. DPT (diphtheria, pertussis and tetanus) vaccines are made this way.

Because each batch of a vaccine originates from different bacteria or viruses growing on different culturing mediums, there will be variations in the characteristics, actions, properties and genetic contaminants in different batches. And this means that some of those batches can cause more problems than others.

Genetic/Bacterial/Viral Contamination

Genetic materials from the tissues on which the viruses/bacteria are grown— plus any viruses or bacteria that may be present in those tissues—can also contaminate a vaccine. Although vaccine manufacturers attempt to screen for contaminants, these screening methods are not foolproof and do *not* detect all possible contaminants.

Historically, one of the worst of these contaminants was the monkey virus known as SV40, which contaminated the very first polio vaccine in 1955. Unfortunately, the problem was not discovered until millions of doses of the vaccine had been given worldwide. It has since been directly related to increased cases of cancer and autoimmune disease in the children and adults who received it.[13]

More recently, one of the world's largest producers of influenza vaccine, Chiron Corporation, was ordered to shut down their vaccine manufacturing plant in Liverpool, England due to "serious and widespread" bacterial contamination throughout the facility.[14] Although the U.S. Food and Drug Administration (FDA) first found contamination problems at the Liverpool plant in 1999 and issued warning letters, it took five years before the British government suspended the plant's license. *Five years of ongoing bacterial contamination* in the world's leading influenza vaccine manufacturing plant!

And that's not all. In December 2007, the giant drug manufacturer Merck Co. recalled 1.2 million doses of their Hib B (Haemophilus influenzae type B) vaccine because of contamination risk due to a sterility problem at their production facility.[15]

And this doesn't address the kinds of contamination that are not being tested for now, and therefore are not removed from vaccines. Nanobacteria, tiny self-replicating bacteria that can be found in the blood of humans and mammals, can cause genetic alteration and abnormal cell growth and proliferation—in other words, cancer.[16] In May 2001, at the 101st general meeting of the American Society for Microbiology, it was disclosed that "... nanobacteria have been found to be a contaminant in previously assumed-to-be-sterile medical products, specifically the IPV Polio Vaccine"[17]

Vaccinations have been routinely injected for decades before anyone had even heard of nanobacterial infection.

The rotavirus vaccine is routinely given to infants at 2, 4 and 6 months of age. This vaccine was first introduced in 1998 and was developed to give protection against the rotavirus, which can create a type of stomach flu with associated fever and diarrhea. This infection is usually self-limiting over the course of a week, and regular allopathic treatment mainly involves managing hydration with ample liquids.

On May 7, 2010 the FDA publicly announced that a porcine circovirus (PCV1), a pig virus, was recently found as a contaminant in GlaxoSmithKline's rotavirus vaccine and that it had been unknowingly present in the vaccine since this version of the vaccine was first developed and introduced in 2008. The FDA told doctors to immediately stop the use of the Rotarix vaccine for rotavirus immunization due to the contamination of this vaccine with the pig virus.

In the same week it was also disclosed that another pig virus, potentially an even more dangerous variety called porcine circovirus type 2 (PCV2), was found as a contaminant in the other rotavirus vaccine given to children, Merck's RotaTeq vaccine.

PCV2 virus causes the following symptoms in infant pigs:

- Wasting and failure to thrive

- Immune suppression

- Respiratory problems

- Kidney, brain and reproductive problems

- Death

What other bacteria, viruses and pathogens are in today's vaccines that we have yet to learn about, that have yet to be identified or that we do not even know how to look for? And how many of these are being unwittingly injected into our children?

The "Hot Batch"

Problematic vaccine batches (those that trigger lots of adverse reactions) are referred to as "hot batches." A "hot batch" either contains a stronger strain of the virus/bacteria or has a higher level of contamination than other batches. This phenomenon has been well-documented in the DPT vaccines, in which "hot batches" have been associated with convulsions, seizures and inflammation of the brain, with associated mood, behavioral and learning disabilities.[18]

Unfortunately, there is no way to determine in advance whether the vaccine you are considering for your child is from a hot batch. This is simply another variable in the "roulette wheel" of vaccinations. The only way you can reduce the possibility of adverse reactions from a hot batch is to give your child additional immune support from the recommended nutritional supplements starting at least one week prior to the vaccination, and continue for at least one month afterward. (See below for specific information on nutritional supplements.)

Additives and Preservatives

In addition to the chemicals used to weaken or deactivate a virus or bacteria, vaccines also contain a long list of other chemicals, additives, stabilizers and preservatives. The most notorious of these is a mercury derivative called thimerosal, which has been used for many years as the primary preservative in many vaccines.

Mercury is one of the most toxic metals on Earth, as our discussions in Chapter 3 showed. It is capable of producing the same toxic effects as lead and arsenic. Studies have documented, for example, that exposure to lead can decrease a child's IQ by up to 10 points. Mercury has the same toxic capacity with the same brain-damaging effects. Ten IQ points is what separates man from the chimpanzee. (The chimpanzee's IQ goes up to 65, and a human's IQ starts at around 75.) This means that these metals can affect and interfere with every aspect of a child's brain, intelligence, learning and development.

For many years, concerned parents and doctors have witnessed changes, including learning disorders and autism, in infants and children, following vaccination. Thimerosal is suspected to be one of the causes of these detrimental and life-altering effects.

Thimerosal has been the focus of worldwide attention, congressional hearings and government inquiries.[19] Yet, even though the U.S. FDA ordered all pharmaceutical companies to stop using it as a preservative in all vaccines in 2000, thimerosal is still found in some influenza vaccines that are routinely recommended and administered to pregnant mothers, infants and children.[20] Some forms of the hepatitis B vaccine also still contain thimerosal.[12, 21]

Other additives and ingredients found in vaccines include:

- Ammonium sulfate

- Latex rubber

- Monosodium glutamate

- Aluminum

- Formaldehyde

- Polysorbate 80

- Glutaraldehyde

- Gentamicin sulfate and polymyxin B

- Neomycin sulfate

- Phenol/phenoxyethanol

- Human and animal cells

- Microorganisms (e.g., nanobacteria)

Individually, each of these additives carries its own toxicity and risk. When they are added together and injected into an infant or child, the toxic burden and risk multiply dramatically. There is no way of knowing in advance which ingredient or ingredients your child may be sensitive to, which makes every vaccination an experiment involving your precious child's body and mind. Each additional vaccination compounds the risk, so it's just a matter of time until your child's immune and nervous systems reach the limit of what they can handle. The toxicity threshold and the number of vaccines that each individual child can endure before adverse consequences begin will depend upon the child's constitutional predisposition, current nutritional status, dietary habits, health history, along with any emotional and environmental stresses.

The Downside of Vaccines

Vaccinations are immunotherapy. The effects they have on the immune system, brain and the neurological system depend on the nature of the vaccine, how it is administered, the ingredients it contains and the "internal terrain" of the child. Among the most common and well-documented consequences of all vaccinations given to children are low-grade encephalitis (inflammation in the brain), seizures, autism, diabetes and rheumatoid arthritis.[22]

In 1986, the U.S. government enacted the National Childhood Vaccine Injury Act, which, among other things, established a fund for compensating the families of children who are injured, maimed or killed by vaccines. The act also created protection for the pharmaceutical companies who manufacture the vaccines by preventing them from being sued directly or bearing legal liability for any injury stemming from a vaccination. Since that time, $1.5 billion have been paid to the children and families of children who were harmed by vaccines. To qualify for this compensation, the adverse effects have to be considered "severe," which are defined as life-threatening illness, prolonged hospitalization, permanent disability or death.[23]

ADMINISTERING VACCINATIONS

We are all exposed to viruses and bacteria on a continual basis, through inhalation or contact with the skin and mucus membranes. And immune cells in these surface "barriers" are well prepared to mount a defense against them. Underneath these surface barriers we also have another series of barrier systems that are at the forefront of our immune system's design and capabilities for containing and protecting against any bacteria or virus that may slip past the first line of defense. We have the intestinal membrane, or immune barrier, to prevent bacteria or viruses that may be in the food we eat from passing out of the intestinal tract and into the rest of our body.

Should the virus or bacteria manage to penetrate deeper into our bodies, other components of our immune systems will be activated: immune scouts, macrophages, T-cells and interferon. All will play a part in the containment, destruction and disposal of the invaders, via a very systematic, methodical and well-orchestrated response.

Our brain even has its own blood/brain barrier comprised of specialized immune cells designed to guard and protect entry into our most precious and vital organ, the brain.

This very effective and sophisticated system of immune membranes, barriers and specialized immune cells has protected human beings for at least 100,000 years. Yet all of these natural systems and stages of defense are completely bypassed, confused and jeopardized when a vaccine is injected past these natural immune barriers and directly into the deeper tissues of the body.

Additionally, it is unheard of for a person to contract measles and mumps or whooping cough and diphtheria simultaneously. When, in nature, would your child be exposed to diptheria, tetanus, pertussis, polio, hepatitis B and influenza all on the same day, within the same minute? Yet that's exactly what happens when a child is given multiple vaccines. When three, four or even six vaccines for such diseases are given during one office visit (e.g., DTaP, polio, Hep B, Hib), they create unprecedented stress and confusion within a young child's immune and detoxification systems. *The risk of detrimental consequences increases exponentially when multiple vaccines are administered routinely and at short intervals.*

Multiple Vaccines in a Single Injection

Multiple vaccinations given in a single injection top the list of the world's worst medical inventions.

Known as "multivalent vaccinations," these include the DTaP (diphtheria, tetanus, pertussis), MMR (measles, mumps, rubella), IPV (polio) and HepB (diphtheria, pertussis, tetanus, polio and hepatitis B), among others. These are not rare or offbeat vaccines; they are commonly administered.

In June 2010, the *Journal of Pediatrics* reported on analysis from the Kaiser Permanente Vaccine Study Center showing that the multivalent vaccine containing measles, mumps, rubella and chickenpox doubles the risk of a fever-related seizure among 1-year-olds and 2-year-olds 7 to 10 days after the shot, compared to giving the MMR vaccine and chickenpox vaccine separately.

The more vaccines injected into your child at the same time, the greater the risk of adverse and negative reactions. More vaccines means more additives, preservatives, contaminants, bacteria and viruses for your child's body, brain and immune system to deal with all at once. And, because their immune systems and brain are still "under construction," still developing, they are most susceptible to adverse effects from the deluge of additives and immune-tampering materials contained in all vaccines.

In spite of this, the standard immunization schedule in the United States recommends that at the ages of 2 and 4 months, infants should be injected with DTaP or DTaP, IPV, HepB shots, each containing three to five different vaccines. In addition, Hib (Haemophilus influenzae) and PCV (pnemococcal) are to be given at the same time, during the same office visit. This makes a total of *seven vaccines given at the same time to a 2-month-old baby*!

How can anyone honestly believe that injecting a 2-month, 4-month or 12-month-old baby with all of these vaccines— containing additives, chemicals, metals, contaminants and bacterial and viral material—can be completely safe? At best, we can say that each child will handle them differently, depending on his or her current nutritional status, immune strength, environmental stress level, toxic load level and constitutional vulnerabilities. At worst, we must recognize that all children will be affected by this onslaught to some degree, in some manner, for the rest of their lives.

At 12 to 15 months of age, the recommended schedule calls for an infant to be injected with MMR, IPV, Hib, DTaP, Hep B, varicella and influenza. *A total of 11 vaccines injected directly into your infant, all at the same time, at the extremely young and delicate age of 12 months*!

Frequency of Administration

Considering the many components, additives and possible contaminants that are contained in vaccines, it's easy to understand how the cumulative effect of repeated doses given in close proximity can stress an infant or child's immune system and detoxification capacity. Each child will have a different level of tolerance that cannot be predicted in advance. Once that threshold has been reached and exceeded, a child's immune system will be unable to respond appropriately and adverse reactions will begin to appear.

This is why the frequency of vaccine administration is a very important consideration. If you do choose to give your child some of the vaccines, then spacing vaccinations further apart will give your child's immune system a chance to recover and prepare for the next challenge or onslaught.

Vaccine ▼ Age ▶	Birth	1 month	2 months	4 months	6 months	12 months	15 months	18 months	24 months	4–6 years	11–12 years	13–14 years	15 years	16–18 years
Hepatitis B¹	HepB	HepB	HepB¹		HepB						HepB Series			
Diphtheria, Tetanus, Pertussis²			DTaP	DTaP	DTaP		DTaP			DTaP	Tdap		Tdap	
Haemophilus influenzae type b³			Hib	Hib	Hib³	Hib								
Inactivated Poliovirus			IPV	IPV		IPV				IPV				
Measles, Mumps, Rubella⁴						MMR				MMR			MMR	
Varicella⁵						Varicella					Varicella			
Meningococcal⁶							Vaccines within broken line are for selected populations				MCV4		MCV4	
											MPSV4		MCV4	
Pneumococcal⁷			PCV	PCV	PCV	PCV			PCV		PPV			
Influenza⁸						Influenza (Yearly)				Influenza (Yearly)				
Hepatitis A⁹									HepA Series					

Recommended Childhood and Adolescent Immunization Schedule UNITED STATES • 2006

DEPARTMENT OF HEALTH AND HUMAN SERVICES • CENTERS FOR DISEASE CONTROL AND PREVENTION

Center for Disease Control and Prevention.
Online at http://www.immunize.org/cdc/child-schedule.pdf

Total Number of Vaccines Given

If a child were to get all of the vaccines listed on the Recommended Childhood and Adolescent Immunization Schedule, he or she would receive an average of 32 vaccinations by the age of 2 years, and a total of 43 vaccinations by 5 years of age! A quarter-century ago, only 11 vaccinations were given by the age of 5, and 50 years ago, just 5 vaccines were given.[24]

Has this huge increase in vaccinations resulted in healthier children? Are children healthier today than 50 years ago? Fifty years ago, 1 in every 50 American children suffered from some form of chronic medical disease. Today, 1 out of every 5 American children suffers from some type of lifelong chronic medical disorder.[25]

One child may be able to handle 10 or 20 vaccines without an overt adverse reaction. For another child, the threshold number may be five, two or even zero. Unfortunately, there is no way to determine this beforehand. With the dramatic increase in the number of vaccines and the frequency of administration over the past years, there is an ever-increasing risk of adverse reactions. It is simply a matter of numbers: more vaccines administered in close proximity will increase the odds that your child's body, immune, brain and nervous system will be overwhelmed by the ongoing barrage at some point. Seizures, low-grade toxic encephalitis (inflammation of the brain), ADD, ADHD, autism and other learning or behavioral problems are all conditions that have been linked to the toxic accumulation and inflammatory effects of the ingredients contained in vaccines.

SHOULD YOU ALLOW YOUR CHILD TO BE VACCINATED?

My personal advice is no and the best advice I can give you is to educate yourself on this subject as much as possible, and then make an informed decision. Don't forget to consider the following:

Successful Treatment

My son Luukas seemed normal—walking at 10 months and saying his first words. He was animated and engaged with the world. His smile was a joy each morning and I was settling into motherhood.

At 1 month Luukas was hospitalized with a urinary tract infection that we learned was a result of a birth defect causing kidney reflux. He was placed on daily doses of antibiotics indefinitely. In addition to the antibiotics, he was getting all the recommended vaccinations. At 1 year, he received his vaccinations, which included more than just the MMR. He also received the polio and chickenpox vaccines that day. Within weeks of turning 1 year old, Luukas deteriorated. He lost his motor coordination, lost all words, lost all eye contact and started throwing long, violent tantrums that would last

---

hours. We were kicked out of every Mommy and Me class, and it was very clear that Luukas was no longer like other kids his age. Venturing out of the house was practically impossible without incident and we became reclusive.

Luukas seemed incapable of handling change of any sort. He would freak out if he spilled anything, or his shirt became wet. He refused to touch sand or put his feet in it. He became rigid in terms of routine and it was like living with a crazy person. Tantrums for not seeing the syrup poured on his waffles, even though the syrup was there. But most painful of all was the loss of his inner spirit and all joy, connection and love that had been there. I missed the little boy I had in the beginning, full of life and connected to the world.

After being kicked out of preschool, and then after Luukas broke my nose during a tantrum, I reached my limit and went for help, thinking that I had failed as a mother. The psychologist suggested I have Luukas developmentally evaluated so she could properly help me. I was not prepared for his diagnosis of autism from UCLA Medical Center, but with a diagnosis, I had information. I was exhausted by the insanity we had been living with, and I was worried about my son's future and his ability to have a childhood and grow into a functioning adult. With the diagnosis I went to work reading, going to lectures and going to conferences. I tried to find out if there was anything that would work or improve our quality of life—for both him and me.

First, I found the association Defeat Autism Now. I began trying different vitamins that I had heard worked for different things, like vitamin A for eye contact, dimethylglycine for vocabulary and speech. I tried the gluten-free/casein-free diet. I started seeing little changes, a few more words and slightly better focus and eye contact... so I wanted to try everything.

I felt the vitamins and supplements were getting out of hand and there was more going on with Luukas' biochemistry than I could handle. Luukas went through a yeast die-off on the gluten-free diet that was something to reckon with. I was feeling overwhelmed that I was on the verge of mixing the wrong vitamins, or that I could potentially make things worse. At that moment, I was given Dr. Murray Clarke's name. Little did I know that he would impact our lives in such a huge and dramatic way.

Luukas began seeing Dr. Clarke at the age of 3. Luukas is 13 today and we still rely on the expertise of Dr. Clarke. Over the years, we realized that Luukas was heavy-metal toxic. We started dealing with the yeast problem, implementing a strict diet, streamlining the daily vitamins, and we started heavy metal chelation. After the first chelation treatment, Luukas seemed dramatically better—like miracle stuff. He was speaking words and calmly drawing pictures. He looked at me and said "Momma, dinosaur," holding up his creation. I cried on my kitchen floor and thanked God. The interventions started working. The speech therapy, occupational therapy, socialization classes, shadow teacher and behavior specialists all contributed. At the age of 8 he was presented at the DAN! Convention as one of the first children "recovered" from autism.

Luukas STILL chelates at least once a year and is on a strict regimen of supplements, which are carefully crafted from lab work overseen by Dr. Clarke. Luukas is amazing. He has friends and has had a girlfriend. Luukas is an INCREDIBLE athlete and quarterback for his football team. He trains year-round with a private quarterback coach and has high hopes for himself in the NFL. He is a high honor roll student in class and has just been accepted into the honors program at a magnet school. He is funny, loving, and has a chance at a bright future.

Those doctors who evaluated him in the early years said he would be in an assisted living center as an adult. They said he would never have a sense of humor, that he would never have friends. There were days I didn't think so either. There were days when Luukas was incapable of entering Dr. Clarke's office, and Dr. Clarke patiently and calmly sat on the floor in the hallway by the elevator to meet us and have our appointment. His patience and kindness have gotten us through illness, breakdowns, regressions and most of all, he's gotten us here to this amazing place we are today. Luukas has a life of hope.

It's clear our environment has changed, that what we eat has changed, and most of all how our society deals with health in general, needs to change. Luukas eats organic foods, takes LOTS of supplements, and he has not been vaccinated again. I have taken control of Luukas' immune system with the help of Dr. Clarke and I take that responsibility very seriously. Homeopathy works. Luukas has not taken antibiotics again since he was 3. It takes trust, patience and diligence to take control of one's health.

Autism is treatable. My son has an opportunity for life now. The diligence and hard work—and of course the expense of it—WORTH IT! I had to look past just getting through a day at school, getting through a play date, getting through a trip to the park. Luukas' health was so much more... it was giving him a chance at life, of having love, of being capable of an intimate relationship one day, holding a job, being a participant in society. Those are the goals that get you through the hard days, the work it took to have him take cod liver oil day after day, and choosing to pay for vitamins instead of other things. I'm here to tell you its all worth it. Seeing my son throw the winning touchdown (against all odds) and the joy on his face—worth it!

- What is the current overall state of your child's health?

- How many times has he or she been given antibiotics?

- How many vaccines has he or she already received?

- What is his or her nutritional status?

- Are there any other stresses that may be affecting him or her, such as new siblings, stressed parents or a recent move?

- Is there a family history on either parent's side of any neurological or autoimmune disorders such as type 1 diabetes, rheumatoid arthritis, Hashimoto's thyroid disease, multiple sclerosis, Alzheimer's or Parkinson's disease?

All of these factors will determine your child's current level of immune strength and vulnerability, to help you gauge how susceptible he or she may be to reacting adversely to a vaccination.

But If You Decide to Vaccinate

If you do decide to give your child some or all of the vaccines, my advice is as follows:

- *Never give a multivalent vaccine.* Separate each vaccine, and only allow one vaccine at a time to be administered. For example, use Mumpsvax, the single antigen vaccine for measles, instead of the multivalent combination vaccine of MMR. Insist that your pediatrician divide each vaccine into separate doses: M (measles), M (mumps) and R (rubella) vaccinations, each to be given individually, with at least three months between each vaccine.

- *Never allow your child to receive a vaccine that contains thimerosal.* (This preservative is found, for example, in some of the influenza vaccines and some hep B vaccines.) Ask your doctor to check and ensure that any hepatitis B and/or influenza vaccine administered to your child does not contain any thimerosal.

- *Never allow your child to receive a vaccine if he or she is suffering from or just getting over an acute infection* (e.g. cold, cough, flu or ear infection). An already burdened immune system should not be subjected to further stress.

- *Be aware that the hep B, MMR, and Rotavirus vaccines have the highest incidence of documented adverse effects and reactions.* You may want to skip these altogether.

- *Consider omitting vaccinations for non-life-threatening infections.* Chickenpox, measles, rubella (German measles), mumps and flu were all considered normal childhood diseases until relatively recently. Nothing has changed; they are still typically not life threatening, especially if treated correctly with homeopathic and naturopathic remedies.

- *Consider your family history.* A family history of neurological disorders such as seizures, Parkinson's disease, dementia, or Alzheimer's disease, or immune disorders such as rheumatoid arthritis, lupus, chronic allergies, multiple sclerosis or diabetes, may make your child more susceptible to an adverse reaction to vaccinations. Be extra careful about giving your child vaccines if there is a family history of any of the above disorders.

- *Give your child extra nutritional support at least 1 week prior and for 1 month following any vaccination.* The support should include the following supplements: vitamin C, colostrum, probiotics, vitamin D and cod liver oil.

  ### Daily Dosages:

  Up to 1 year of age: vitamin C, 250 mg; colostrum, ½ teaspoon; probiotics, ¼ teaspoon; vitamin D, 400 iu; cod liver oil, ½ teaspoon

  2-4 years: vitamin C, 500mg; colostrum, ½ teaspoon; probiotics, ¼ teaspoon; vitamin D, 800 iu; cod liver oil, 1 teaspoon

  5-8 years: vitamin C, 1000 mg; colostrum, 1 teaspoon; probiotics, ½ teaspoon; vitamin D, 1,000 iu; cod liver oil, 1 teaspoon

- *Allow at least three months' time between each vaccination to ensure detoxification and recovery.* Give your child's body, brain and immune system time to detoxify, recover and regroup between vaccinations. Three months is the minimum time for this process.

- *Homeopathic and osteopathic support.* It is recommended to give your child their homeopathic constitutional remedy and osteopathic treatments during this time as suggested by your naturopathic, homeopathic or osteopathic health-care practitioner.

Wait Before You Vaccinate

When parents ask me what age I think is best to start giving a child vaccinations, I usually say, "When he or she turns 100." However, if you do decide to vaccinate your children, remember that the longer you wait, the stronger your child's immune and detoxification systems will become, and the better he or she will be able to handle the inflammatory and immune reactions that vaccines create. For this reason, I suggest that no vaccinations be given until at least age 2.

Why Wait Until Age 2?

A full 80 percent of the brain's growth occurs within the first two years of life[26], and it is exceedingly important that nothing interfere with its development during this time. Because the brain is so important, it has its own immune cells and system, which operates independently from the rest of the body. The special immune cells found in the brain (known as microglia and astrocytes) are an important part of the blood-brain barrier and will react to each and every vaccine.[27] Russell Blaylock, M.D., a neurologist and neurosurgeon, published an extremely well-referenced article documenting exactly how vaccinations provoke an inflammatory immune response within the brain, complete with a cascade of toxic cytokines, excitotoxins, arachidonic acid and chemokines.[28] All of these substances are normal components of a short-term immune response, but when vaccines are given together or in close proximity and are frequently repeated, this inflammatory immune response can escalate, accumulate and continually aggravate the brain. This prolonged inflammation then drastically interferes with the proper growth, development and function of the child's brain.

Severe reactions result in autism, with the degree of brain dysfunction ranging all along the autistic spectrum. Medium reactions may lead to mood or behavioral disorders or other types of learning disorders like ADD or ADHD. If the vaccination(s) should harm the immune system more than the brain, your child may develop allergies, eczema, become more prone to catching colds, coughs, flu and ear infections, or suffer from autoimmune disorders such as diabetes and rheumatoid arthritis.[29]

You are courting danger and exponentially increasing the risk of adverse reactions and obstructions to brain growth and development if you allow your child to receive any vaccination before the age of 2. If you do choose to vaccinate your child with some or all of the vaccines, wait until he or she is at least 2 if not 3 years old.

It's Your Choice

To vaccinate or not to vaccinate is one of the biggest health decisions you'll ever make for your child. It is your constitutional, philosophical, spiritual and religious right to do what you think is best. Vaccinations are not compulsory, so don't allow your pediatrician, school, family or community to bully you into vaccinating your child if you feel it isn't right. Take the time to educate yourself and consider your options. Almost every state in America acknowledges that every parent has a constitutional and philosophical right to decide whether they want their child to be vaccinated or not.

Be aware that guilt is a powerful factor in the vaccination world. Pediatricians and school officials often tell parents that if they do not vaccinate, they are placing other children and the community at an unfair risk. This is untrue. If other parents choose to vaccinate their children, then they have no reason to fear risk of disease from an unvaccinated child because their child should not be able to contract those diseases.

The vaccination decision is in your hands. Decide what makes you most comfortable and proceed from there, on your own terms.

Note: A detailed discussion of each of the most common vaccines currently in use, plus a risk assessment, can be found in Appendix II: Rating the Vaccines.

Chapter 6

Optimal Health: Pre-Conception

The excellence of the fruit depends upon the health of the tree from which it springs, and the health of the tree is dependent upon the quality of the earth in which it grew. We humans are not so different than the tree: the health of a newborn baby reflects the quality of the parents' sperm and egg at the time of conception, plus the mother's health and circumstances during pregnancy. Common sense tells us that if both mother and father are healthy and vital, the mother's nutrition is optimal and the environment she lives in is nourishing and enjoyable, the baby who grows within her should also enjoy radiant health.

Creating another human being and bringing that person into this world is surely one of the greatest endeavors anyone can undertake. And since all of the world's great accomplishments begin with a thought, and then with a plan followed by preparation, continued action and effort, it makes perfect sense that all prospective parents should plan, prepare and live in ways that ensure the best possible health for their baby. And the time to engage in such planning and preparation is *before* conception occurs, during the period I call pre-conception.

It is no longer debatable whether a woman's exposure to pollutants and the toxins accumulated during pregnancy will affect the health, development and intelligence of the newborn baby. It is an unassailable fact. In a landmark study published in the August 2009 issue of the *Journal of Pediatrics*, researchers conclusively linked air pollution exposure before birth with lower IQ scores in childhood. The children of the mothers exposed to the most pollution before birth scored on average four to five IQ points lower than children with less exposure.[1]

Recent studies from Russia show that an alarming 50 percent of Russian children are now born with some type of birth defect or physical developmental disorder, both of which can be linked to the disastrous levels of environmental contamination in that country.[2]

Forty years ago, 1 in 50 children in the United States grew up with and suffered from some type of chronic illness for lifetime. Now, that number is 1 in every 5 children. Exposure to environmental pollutants and toxins is one of the biggest factors contributing to the extraordinary increase in the number of sick children.[3, 4]

In light of such research, the only conscientious choice for parents-to-be is to detoxify as much as possible *before* conception, then neutralize any exposure to toxins that occurs throughout pregnancy. In this way you can be sure that you are offering your child the best possible foundation for excellent health, in spite of the polluted environment that surrounds all of us.

A NEW LIFE BEGINS

When sperm meets an egg, a miracle occurs: the beginning of

a new life. The most important stage of the embryo's growth is "gastrulation," a phase that takes place during the eight weeks immediately following conception. During this critical stage, the mass of new cells created since conception separates into three distinct layers, each of which will give rise to specific tissues, organs and systems. The outer layer produces cells that form the skin and nervous system; the inner layer produces cells that form the lining of the digestive system and associated organs like the liver, while the middle layer produces cells that form the heart, kidneys, genitals, bones, muscles and blood. By the 22nd day post-conception, the heart has begun to beat.

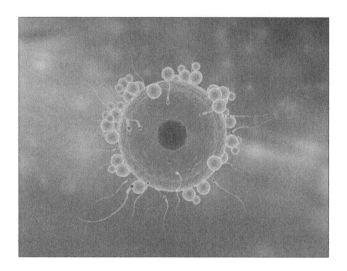

Within six to eight weeks after conception, the basic template for the body has been constructed. What is created during this time will determine the form, development and outcome of all further physical growth for this person, as a baby, child and adult. At six to seven weeks, the beginning of arms and legs can be seen, and neurons (brain cells), multiplying at the rate of 100,000 cells per hour, build the brain. By eight weeks following conception, the baby's brain, face, liver, kidneys, lungs and digestive system are recognizable and the embryo becomes a fetus.[5] The initial "constitution" has now been established and set: the foundation has been laid.

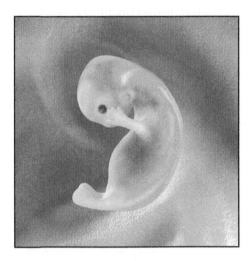

When building a house, the foundation is the most important part: it determines the shape, size and integrity of the rest of the structure. The same is true for a developing baby. All further growth is determined by and built upon the foundation that has been made during the eight-week period of gastrulation.[6] Thus, whether mother-to-be or father-to-be, the importance of preparing yourself physically and emotionally prior to conception simply can't be overstated. This can be best accomplished through the following means:

- proper diet

- detoxification through vitamins, minerals, antioxidants, amino acids, nutraceuticals (natural substances found in food that have medicinal properties to treat or prevent certain diseases) and sauna

- supplementation with prenatal vitamin/mineral formulas, omega-3 and omega-6 oils and probiotics

- adjusting and aligning your body with osteopathy

- balancing your body, mind and soul with a homeopathic "constitutional" remedy

In short: eat well, detoxify, supplement, get clean, get healthy, strengthen ... *then* get pregnant.

PRE-CONCEPTION DIET

The food you eat on a daily basis is the single most important physical factor in determining whether you'll be radiantly healthy or inclined toward illness. So, when setting the stage for a healthy pregnancy and healthy baby, look first to your dietary habits.

Eat Organic Foods

First and foremost, eat organic foods whenever possible. Your food is meant to deliver nutrients and nourishment, not chemicals in the form of pesticides, herbicides, hormones and antibiotics. By definition, organic foods—including fruits, vegetables, meats, poultry and dairy products— contain none of these. Consider buying produce from local farmers markets where you can find organic and locally grown fresh fruits and vegetables. (There is a lot of truth to that old saying, "Know your farmer, know your food....") Organic foods are also available at health food stores. The U. S. Department of Agriculture (USDA) oversees the certification of organic foods and produce in America. Reputable stores should be adhering to USDA or the applicable country's guidelines and supplying only organic foods that have been certified.

Follow the Blood Type Diet

It's important that you eat the foods that particularly suit you by following the Blood Type Diet. (*See* Chapter 1: Dietary Problems and Solutions.) This will ensure that you are eating the foods that are the most easily digested, metabolized and absorbed by your body. These foods will also help reduce the burden placed on your immune system. Following the blood type diet during pregnancy will help you stay healthier and stronger, which should translate to a healthier and stronger baby.

Avoid the NonKosher Foods

I also suggest that you follow the recommendations of the oldest and original dietary food guide—the Torah—and eat kosher food. Although associated in most people's minds with Judaism, kosher foods and dietary guidelines were designed specifically to create and maintain good health. The most important directives of kosher dietary rules, in my opinion, are as follows:

Avoid pork

Of all animals, the flesh of the pig is the most similar in protein structure to that of humans. Because of this, pig flesh harbors viruses that can easily penetrate our bodies, adapt to our protein structure and slip by our immune systems, unnoticed and unchecked.[7] In addition, the pig is one of the few animals that will eat its own fecal matter. The dirt, energy and substance of the feces ends up in the pig's flesh, which then ends up in you if you eat pork.

Notably, according to the Blood Type Diet, pork is the only meat that doesn't test well and is not recommended for *any* blood type.

Avoid fish that do not have scales or fins

Just by avoiding fish without scales and fins you will be excluding the most polluted fish documented by today's science. Fish that do not have scales or fins include shark, swordfish, squid, eel, flounder, sole and catfish. Of all of the fish in the ocean, shark and swordfish have been shown to contain the highest levels of mercury. This is because they are at the top of the food chain, tend to live a long time and over their lifetime accumulate mercury by eating other smaller, mercury-laden fish. Because of the amount of mercury found in shark and swordfish these days, the U.S. Food and Drug Administration has advised pregnant women and children to **never** eat shark or swordfish.[8]

Fish that have no scales or fins and are bottom-dwellers are also problematic because they exist at the bottom of the food chain and survive by eating the rubbish, debris and fecal matter of other fish. These fish include catfish, flounder, eel and sole.

Avoid shellfish and crustaceans

This category includes lobster, crab, shrimp, oysters, mussels, scallops and clams. Shellfish and crustaceans dwell primarily on the ocean floor and, like the bottom-dwelling fish, live off the rubbish, debris and fecal matter of the sea's ecosystem. Recent studies show that the pollutants infesting the world's oceans (PCBs, dioxins, insecticides, phosphate fertilizers, plastics, and pharmaceutical drugs) are now found in the highest concentrations in these bottom-dwelling shellfish and crustaceans.[9] Shellfish also contain high levels of problematic bacteria and viruses, including *Vibrio vulnificus, Yersinia enterocolitica,* and *Fecal coliform*[10], which then place a greater burden on your immune system.

By following these kosher guidelines, you will automatically screen out and avoid the foods that contain the highest degree of pollutants, along with the greatest amounts of bacterial, viral and fecal contamination. These guidelines are recommended not only during the pre-conception period, but forever after.

Relax and Enjoy Your Meals!

By integrating organic foods, avoiding the non-kosher food groups and selecting the foods that best suit your blood type, you now have created the cleanest and healthiest diet possible for you. Now, it is time to sit back, relax and eat your food in an **enjoyable and peaceful** manner. Chew your food thoroughly and eat slowly to ensure the proper digestion of the food nutrients. Avoid working, stressful conversations or watching TV while you eat. Instead, embrace and enjoy every bite of that tasty organic meal! Eating should be a wonderful and relaxing experience.

PRENATAL SUPPLEMENTS

During conception and pregnancy, your body needs a wide array of foods and nutrients, not only to keep itself healthy and strong but to create another human being. The foundation of a healthy diet will always start with each meal containing well-balanced proportions of **protein** (meat, poultry, fish, eggs, cheese), **carbohydrates** (noodles, pasta and bread—ideally all gluten free—rice, vegetables, fruit), and **fats and oils** (olive oil, flaxseed oil, butter, coconut oil). In addition, the demand for all the "essential" nutrients (vitamins, minerals, essential fatty acids and amino acids) increases and is of utmost importance during this time.

A high-quality prenatal vitamin/mineral supplement and cod liver oil can supply all of the necessary vitamins, minerals and omega-3 essential fatty acids. In addition, take extra vitamin C to support your immune system and help protect your body from environmental pollutants. Then, by eating a well-balanced diet, which includes plenty of complex carbohydrates and some form of protein at each meal, you should be able to obtain all of the nutrients that you need.

Ideally, for at least three months prior to conception, the mother-to-be should take:

- *A high-quality prenatal vitamin/mineral* – High-quality means that all the vitamins are in their natural form (e.g., vitamin E is in the form of d-alpha tocopherol, (not dl-alpha tocopherol). Minerals should be in chelated form for optimum absorption (e.g., calcium citrate rather than calcium carbonate). High-quality also means that there are absolutely no artificial additives such as artificial colorings or flavorings.

  Dosage: Follow the suggested dosage on label and take with meals.

- *Cod liver oil* — To ensure that you and your baby will have all the omega-3 fatty acids and DHA that are required for a healthy pregnancy. The product label should always state that it's certified to be completely free of any mercury, PCBs or dioxins.

  If the label does not state that the oil is free of these contaminants, do not buy it.

  Dosage: One tablespoon or three 1,000 mg capsules daily with meals.

- *Vitamin C* — In addition to the vitamin C contained in your prenatal vitamin (usually around 200 mg), take 1,000 mg of vitamin C twice daily. This extra vitamin C supports your immune system, and can make you less susceptible to infections during your pregnancy. Vitamin C is also the primary antioxidant for assisting your body in gently neutralizing, detoxifying and eliminating metals (mercury, lead, arsenic) and other chemical pollutants.

Dosage: 1,000 mg twice daily with meals.

For at least 3 months prior to conception, the father-to-be should take:

- *A high-quality multivitamin/mineral* – many quality companies now have multivitamin formulas developed specifically for men. See your local health food store.

  Dosage: Follow suggested dosage on label, take with meals.

- *Cod liver oil* – The omega-3 fatty acids can help make every man healthier. The product label should always state that it's certified to be completely free of any mercury, PCBs or dioxin.

  Dosage: 1 tablespoon or three 1,000 mg capsules daily.

- *Extra vitamin C* — To neutralize, detoxify and eliminate metals (mercury, lead, arsenic) and other chemical pollutants. To create healthier sperm.

  Dosage: 1,000 mg twice daily with meals.

PRE-CONCEPTION DETOXIFICATION

Detoxifying and cleansing the body prior to conception can be an important part of preparing the body for pregnancy. Detoxification involves identifying and neutralizing any form of toxin or pollutant, then transporting these substances safely out of the body via the urine or the bile by way of the stool. Most toxins accumulate and are stored in body fat and connective tissues. This is the body's way of putting these potentially harmful substances in "safe storage" and keeping them away from more vital organs like the brain. When you begin the process of detoxification, you'll dislodge and release these accumulated toxins into your bloodstream, lungs, liver and intestines so they can be eliminated. Thus, the level of actively circulating toxins temporarily increases while they are on the way to being eliminated.

If you are already pregnant while detoxifying, then your developing baby may be exposed to this removal and transportation of toxins. **Thus, it is always best to complete the detoxification process** *prior to* **conception and** *not pursue it at all during pregnancy.*

The liver is the primary organ of detoxification and has four main methods for identifying, neutralizing and sending toxic substances out of the body: filtering the blood, bile excretion and Phase I and Phase II detoxification. Additional ways of detoxifying include ingestion of fiber and plenty of water.

Filtering the Blood

Approximately two quarts of blood pass through the liver every minute for detoxification purposes. A healthy liver will be able to filter out over 90 percent of any toxins during this first filtration stage. Most of these toxins will then be funneled into the bile for excretion.

Bile Excretion

Each day the liver produces approximately one quart of bile which is used as a "transport vehicle" for carrying and dumping toxic substances into the intestines, where they will be eliminated through the stool.

Phase I Detoxification

This detox pathway involves a two-step enzymatic process that converts toxic chemicals into less harmful substances that can be safely escorted out of the body. The liver accomplishes this through the use of cytochrome P450 enzymes and the chemical reactions known as oxidation, reduction and hydrolysis.

Phase II Detoxification

Also called the conjugation pathway, during Phase II the liver cells add another substance to the toxic chemical to make it even less harmful. This step also makes the toxins water soluble so the body can excrete them through the bile or urine. Phase II detoxification occurs via the processes of glutathione conjugation, amino acid conjugation, acetylation, glucuronidation, methylation and sulfation.

The liver requires the right amounts of vitamins, minerals, amino acids and antioxidants for each of these detox methods and pathways to work effectively. You can assist in the process by supplementing with the particular nutrients required for each step. The most important nutrients for Phase I are vitamin C, B complex vitamins, vitamin E, selenium, glutathione and alpha-lipoic acid. The most important nutrients for Phase II are cysteine, methionine, glycine, acetyl-CoA, MSM (methylsulfonylmethane), SAMe (S-adenosyl-methionine) and glutathione.

Fiber

After the liver has processed and neutralized any toxins or pollutants, they are placed into the bile and dumped into the intestines. At this point, plenty of fiber is necessary for the speedy transit of these substances through the intestines to ensure that they are completely eliminated with little or no reabsorption. Fiber is found in foods; however, when purposefully detoxifying it is a good idea to use additional dietary fiber in supplement form.

Water

Pure water is essential to flush toxins that have been processed by the liver out of the body through the urine and the intestines.

IDENTIFYING TOXINS IN YOUR BODY

You can identify the quantity and types of harmful substances that have accumulated in your body through the following kinds of tests:

- Metal testing (hair or urine analysis)

- Chemical testing. Samples may be taken of your blood, urine, breast milk or even semen to analyze levels of toxic chemicals. The laboratory that specializes in testing for environmental toxins in the U.S. is Metametrix Lab (www. metametrix.com).

- Digestive and intestinal ecology and function (a comprehensive digestive stool analysis, usually referred to as CDSA test)

- Liver function, kidney function and blood chemistry (comprehensive blood panel)

The beauty of testing is that you can check and retest to monitor the effectiveness of the detoxification process and ensure that these substances have been eliminated from your body *before* you conceive.

Once you obtain this information from your naturopathic, osteopathic or medical doctor, you can focus on the types of toxins that require the most attention and your doctor can prioritize the results and organize an effective detoxification program for you.

I suggest you work directly with a health professional who is well-versed in detoxification methods and can design a detox program specifically for you. Alternatively, you can use the suggestions in the following section to guide you in divesting your body of the complete spectrum of metals and chemicals with this detoxification protocol.

DETOX PROTOCOLS

The following detoxification formulas/protocols should be followed by both the mother-to-be and the father-to-be for at least 3 months prior to conception. Take these formulas 5 days a week, with 2 days off each week to allow the body to process and eliminate the toxins. Be sure to drink ample amounts of pure spring water (at least 4-6 glasses daily) throughout the process. Take dosages of all products according to label instructions.

Warning!

Detoxifying and cleansing the body prior to conception can be an important part of preparing the body for pregnancy. *However, it should only be done before conceiving, not during the pregnancy.* Detoxification during pregnancy carries the risk of exposing the baby to higher levels of toxins.

---

1. Start with *ClearVite by Apex Energetics* for a systemic cleansing and detoxification effect on the digestive system, liver and kidneys.

    Key ingredients:

- Silymarin (milk thistle)

- N-acetyl-L-cysteine

- L- glutamine

- L-lysine

- Glycine

- Probiotics: Lactobacillus acidophilus

- Enzymes: amylase, cellulose, protease

2. After 2 weeks, to work more deeply to detox and eliminate metals and additional chemicals, add

    HM Nano-Detox liquid by Premier Research Lab

    Key Ingredient:

    - Chlorella. This type of sea algae is by far the most effective nutrient for drawing out and eliminating metals (particularly mercury). This product contains chlorella that has been broken down into nano-sized particles, which greatly increases absorption and effectiveness.

    and **Gentle Fibers by Jarrow Formulas**

    Key Ingredients:

    - Fibers/Flavonoids

    - Insoluble fiber (cellulose and hemicellulose)

    - Soluble fiber (pectin, mucilage)

    - Flavonoids (hesperidin, naringen, limictrol)

    - Lignans (from flaxseed meal)

Continue with these 3 formulas for another 2 weeks and

then take 1 week off. Repeating this sequence monthly for 3 months is the ideal way to easily and effectively clean your body of years of accumulated environmental contaminants.

Sauna

Saunas should be utilized prior to conception but *not* during your pregnancy.

The sauna is a wonderful and extremely effective means of helping the body detoxify and eliminate metals and chemicals. The body tends to accumulate and store toxic chemicals in the fatty tissues. Promoting heat within the body allows the release of fat-soluble toxins, which move into the bloodstream where they can be flushed out via perspiration, urine or bile.

Two types of sauna treatments are available these days: the traditional electric version with heated rocks and the newer infra-red sauna. Infra-red saunas create a slightly different kind of heat that warms the body more from the inside out than the outside in. Both types of sauna assist in detoxification, improve circulation through dilation of the blood vessels, and improve immune function by stimulating the release of white blood cells. But the infra-red saunas may be able to promote a more effective detoxification because of their inside-out method of heating the body.

When utilizing the sauna as a part of a detoxification program, spend 15-30 minutes in the sauna every other day for 4-6 weeks. For maintenance, twice weekly is good. Be sure to drink 8 ounces of water with each session and shower immediately afterward to rinse away any toxins in your perspiration and sweat. Also, take your prenatal vitamins and minerals with extra vitamin C to supply the antioxidants your body needs to help neutralize the toxins that are released.

Remember: Do *not* sauna while you are pregnant.

Osteopathy

I highly recommend that you prepare your body for the upcoming changes associated with your pregnancy through osteopathic manipulative techniques (OMT). Osteopathy, the most sophisticated discipline for adjusting and aligning the body, can ensure that all aspects of the brain, nervous system, lymphatic system and internal organs are functioning properly. Not only can osteopathy help prepare you for conception, it can also help you maintain a healthy pregnancy.

A recent study found that women who received osteopathic care throughout pregnancy had lower rates of Cesarean section delivery, pre-term delivery, umbilical cord prolapse and meconium-stained amniotic fluid, compared to women who did not receive this treatment[11].

I strongly suggest that you start treatments at least 2 months prior to conception and follow your osteopath's advice for maintenance treatment throughout your pregnancy.

Homeopathic Constitutional Remedy

Taking the single correct homeopathic remedy can improve your physical, emotional, mental, and most importantly, spiritual health. A well-chosen homeopathic remedy based specifically on your persona, character, nature, life history and life patterns will have a cleansing, strengthening and balancing effect on every level of your being. Find a qualified and well-educated Hahnemannian homeopath to prescribe this remedy. You will find a detailed explanation of homeopathic constitutional remedies in Chapter 4 in the section on homeopathic medicine. Taking this remedy for a minimum of 3-6 months prior to conception and then throughout your pregnancy will have a tremendously positive and lasting effect on you and, especially, your baby.

LAYING THE GROUNDWORK FOR A HEALTHY PREGNANCY

Preparing your body for pregnancy will make the process smoother and healthier for both you and your baby. Detoxification is important, but you must do it *before* conceiving, *not* during pregnancy. Don't get too upset by the amount of pollutants and toxins in our environment: they're an unavoidable part of today's world. Just do as much as possible to avoid these substances, and help your body neutralize, detoxify and eliminate those that you can't avoid.

At the same time that you're detoxifying your body, don't forget to detoxify your home:

- Use only eco-friendly and organic products (such as biologically clean soaps, detergents, laundry powders and household cleaners).

- Use only eco-friendly and organic products on yourself (biologically clean shampoos, toothpaste, creams, cleansers and deodorants).

- Drink pure artesian spring water or purify your water

supply with a high-quality three-step filter.

- Wherever possible, utilize non-toxic furniture, carpets, flooring and bedding.

Remember: Eat well, detoxify, supplement, get clean, get healthy, strengthen ... *then* **get pregnant.**

Chapter 7

Optimal Health: Pregnancy and Birth

Pregnancy is the beginning of an exciting new chapter in your life, and the beginning of another lifetime for your baby's soul. It's the time to focus on nourishment, comfort, security, contentedness and excellent health for both of you. Your health and well-being throughout pregnancy, the health of the father-to-be at conception, the impressions, energy and environment your baby experiences during pregnancy, as well as the destiny of your baby's soul, will all determine the degree of health and the kind of life that your child will ultimately create for himself or herself.

If you were fortunate enough to have completed the recommended pre-conception preparation (see Chapter 6), you are in a very favorable position to give your baby an optimal start in life. However, as we all know, not all pregnancies occur on a planned and timely basis. So if you discover that you are pregnant and haven't gone through the pre-conception preparation, start following the recommendations in this chapter immediately, but *do not* attempt any kind of detoxification. (See the "Detoxification" section of Chapter 6 for a complete explanation.)

As a man, I am far from qualified to write about the state of pregnancy: that is a woman's right only. But I can tell you that based on the experiences of the many mothers-to-be that I have seen in my clinic, the most important areas to address during pregnancy are food and diet, nutritional supplementation, exercise, home environment, osteopathy, homeopathy, acupuncture, and certain herbal, nutritional and homeopathic remedies.

FOOD AND DIET

The food and diet guidelines for pregnancy mirror the ones detailed in Chapters 1 and 6, as summarized below:

Well-Balanced meals with Plenty of Protein

The foundation of a healthy diet will always start with each meal containing well-balanced proportions of **protein** (meat, poultry, fish, eggs, cheese), **carbohydrates** (rice, noodles, pasta, bread, vegetables, fruit), and **fats and oils** (olive oil, flaxseed oil, butter, coconut oil).

Eat Organic Foods

This includes fruits, vegetables, meats, poultry and dairy products that are certified organic, which means they are free of any added pesticides, herbicides, hormones, antibiotics, steroids, artificial colorings or artificial flavorings. Each country has its own organic certification authority, usually conducted through the government's department of agriculture. In the United States, the U. S. Department of Agriculture (USDA) is responsible for overseeing and enforcing these standards. The combination of the USDA requirements and reputable store management should mean that you can trust these certifications.

Follow the Blood Type Diet

Eat the foods that best suit your specific blood type. By following the Blood Type Diet, you can greatly reduce the degree of stress and amount of wear and tear exerted on your digestive and immune systems. Doing so will, among other things, help reduce the likelihood of developing morning sickness, nausea or loss of appetite during your pregnancy.

Eat According to Kosher Law

Remember that the original purpose of kosher law is to help people avoid unclean, unhealthy foods. Non-kosher foods are the animals, fish and shellfish that innately carry the highest levels of bacterial, viral, fecal and environmental contamination due to their position in the food chain and the kinds of matter they ingest.[1] As such, you should avoid the following:

- pork[2]

- fish that do not have scales or fins (such as shark, swordfish, eel, sole, flounder and catfish)

- shellfish and crustaceans (including lobster, crab, shrimp, oysters, mussels, scallops and clams)[3]

Avoiding these foods will reduce your exposure (and that of your baby) to many types of bacteria, viruses and toxins.

Avoid Fish with the Highest Amount of Mercury

Because of the amount of mercury found in shark and swordfish these days, the U.S. Food and Drug Administration has advised women **never** to eat shark or swordfish during pregnancy. The same guidelines also recommend reducing tuna consumption to 6 ounces per week for albacore, and 12 ounces per week for "total variety of fish, including light canned tuna."[4]

Larger "predator" fish tend to accumulate mercury at higher levels than smaller fish, who feed more on vegetation than other fish and who do not have as long of a lifespan as the larger fish.[5]

My advice to women and mothers is to choose the fish that are the least contaminated from mercury and PCBs, which are salmon, trout, sardines, herring, pilchard, snapper, cod and mahi-mahi. Always buy "wild caught" to avoid the residues of antibiotics and other drug treatments that farmed fish are exposed to.[6]

Relax and Enjoy Your Meals!

Eat your meals in a peaceful, enjoyable and healthful manner whenever possible to fully receive all nutritional benefits.

In addition:

Drink Clean, Pure Water

Every day, drink at least four 8-ounce glasses of pure, clean, artesian spring water or extremely well-filtered tap water. An excellent water filtration system should always include at least three filtration stages: carbon pre-filter, reverse osmosis and a carbon post-filter.

NUTRITIONAL SUPPLEMENTATION

The requirement for all the "essential" nutrients (vitamins, minerals, essential fatty acids and amino acids) increases and is of utmost importance during pregnancy. Nutrients provide the building blocks for your baby's growth and development. The "essential nutrients" consist of the vitamins, minerals, omega-3 and omega-6 fatty acids, and amino acids that play a critical role in the vast array of metabolic functions that power the body (especially during pregnancy).[7]

Vitamins

Vitamins A, B1, B2, B3, B5, B6, B12; folic acid; biotin; vitamins C, D, E; choline; vitamin K

Minerals

Calcium, magnesium, sodium, potassium, copper, iron, manganese, chromium, selenium, sulfur, iodine, fluorine, molybdenum, silicon, cobalt, tin, nickel, vanadium, phosphorous, chlorine, zinc

Amino Acids

Arginine, histidine, leucine, isoleucine, lysine, methionine,

phenylalanine, threonine, tryptophan, valine

Fatty Acids

Omega-3 (linoleic acid), omega-6 (linolenic acid)

These 14 vitamins, 21 minerals, 2 fatty acids and 10 amino acids create the complete spectrum of essential nutrients, each with its own function, and yet designed to work collectively with others to accomplish all of the necessary metabolic tasks.

The importance of these nutrients increases from the moment of conception and continues as the baby grows in the womb. Deficiencies in certain nutrients can have dire results. For example, a folic acid deficiency increases the risk of neural tube defects, which can result in spina bifida, a condition in which part of the spinal cord is exposed and malformed. This usually leads to some form of paralysis, fluid accumulation in the brain and associated physical and mental developmental problems. A calcium deficiency can increase the risk of pre-eclampsia, a condition which produces elevated blood pressure with inflammation during pregnancy, and eclampsia, in which convulsions and seizures during pregnancy accompany the high blood pressure. Conversely, current studies have documented the many benefits gained by both mother and baby when nutritional supplements are used during pregnancy, including improved birth weight, reduced risk of premature births and better overall health.[8, 9]

In light of this knowledge, the following nutritional supplements should be taken on a daily basis throughout the pregnancy:

Prenatal Multivitamin/Mineral

Take a high-quality prenatal multivitamin/mineral daily throughout pregnancy. A health-enhancing formula will provide all of the essential vitamins, plus the primary minerals (calcium, magnesium, copper, iron, manganese, chromium, selenium, iodine, phosphorous, zinc). Make sure it does not contain any artificial colorings or flavorings, which are completely unnecessary and potentially harmful.

Supplementing daily can contribute to

- a reduced risk of birth defects, including neural tube defects, cardiovascular defects, limb deformities, urinary tract defects and hydrocephalus (accumulation of fluid on the brain)[9, 10]

- increased birth weight and lower risk of pre-term delivery[11]

- improved immune strength, plus antioxidant protection from environmental pollutants[12, 13]

Omega-3 Fatty Acids

Omega-3s derived from fish oils contain high levels of DHA (docosahexanoic acid), which is the main nutrient required for proper brain function and brain growth. During the third trimester, a mother may lose 3 percent of her brain mass as she transfers DHA to her baby. This is sometimes noticed as a decrease in memory or absent-mindedness. At six weeks postpartum, the levels of DHA in a new mother are often substantially lower than levels in non-pregnant women[14], which can contribute to further decreases in memory, plus mood disturbances. Researchers have found low levels of DHA in the breast milk and red blood cells of mothers suffering from postpartum depression[15], which is not good for either mother or baby. However, with omega-3 supplementation during pregnancy, you can ensure that your baby receives what he or she needs for proper brain growth, while preventing postpartum depression and memory problems for yourself.

Studies show that supplementation with omega-3 oils can also reduce the risk of pre-term delivery[16], promote an easier birth, aid in eye development and improve your baby's IQ.[17] For all of these reasons, omega-3 supplements are recommended throughout pregnancy. Cod liver oil is a great source for these omega-3s.

Dosage: 1 tablespoon or three 1,000 mg capsules daily (with meals) of omega-3 fatty acids. Absolutely insist that the omega3 supplement you use is certified be free of mercury, PCBs and dioxins, and that this is stated on the label.

Calcium and Magnesium

Calcium plays a crucial part in the growth and development of your baby's skeletal system and is also intimately involved in the conduction of nerve impulses, as well as muscle, heart and arterial function. Thanks to its wide-ranging functions, calcium can treat and prevent pre-eclampsia and eclampsia.[18] The U.S. FDA recommends 1,000 mg of calcium daily during pregnancy. Doses of up to 2,000 mg have been effective in treating pre-eclampsia and eclampsia.[19]

Dosage: Up to 1,000 mg daily with meals. The calcium should be in the form of calcium citrate along with the magnesium as magnesium citrate, for best absorption. Calcium should always be taken with magnesium for optimal absorption and effects in a 2:1 ratio of calcium to magnesium (e.g., 1,000 mg calcium to 500 mg magnesium).

Vitamin C

Higher blood levels of vitamin C in pregnant mothers have been correlated with increased baby weight and height, both at birth and after birth.[20, 21] In addition, studies have demonstrated vitamin C's ability to protect fetuses from harm caused by environmental toxins and metals.[22] This is a huge benefit in this day and age. Protecting your baby from the toxicity and harmful effects of chemicals and metals during pregnancy will reduce the risk of birth defects, developmental disorders and autism. I recommend taking an additional 1,000 mg of vitamin C twice daily, above and beyond the amount found in your prenatal vitamin (typically about 200mg). This provides maximum antioxidant effects and environmental protection.

Dosage: 1,000 mg twice daily with meals, in addition to the amount found in your prenatal vitamin.

Probiotics

The intestines are an ecosystem unto themselves. "Probiotics" refers to several species of "friendly bacteria" that live within the intestines and establish the foundation for a healthy digestive and immune system. By maintaining a healthy ecosystem in the digestive tract, the probiotic bacteria automatically help eliminate unwanted ("unfriendly") bacteria, viruses, yeast and fungi.[23] When the "good" bacteria keep the "bad" bugs from taking up residence in the intestines, your immune strength, digestion, absorption and elimination are all improved. Probiotics are also actively involved in the metabolism of essential nutrients, particularly aiding metabolization and absorption of the B-vitamin family, including biotin, folic acid, niacin, pantothenic acid, riboflavin, thiamin, vitamins B6, B12 and K.[24]

Supplementing your diet during pregnancy with probiotics transfers the following benefits to your baby:

- improved immune viral defense through the increase of interleukin and interferon gamma release (immune factors made by the immune system to attack and eliminate viruses)[25]

- improved immune function reducing the incidence of allergies in the newborn[26]

- reduced incidence of eczema in newborn babies and infants[27]

- improved intestinal colonization of the probiotic bacteria in the newborn, resulting in improved immune function and digestion[28]

- reduced incidence of digestive and gastrointestinal disorders in both mother and baby[29]

- healthier levels of omega-3 fatty acids in the placenta, providing more nourishment for the growing fetus

Ideally, your probiotic supplement should contain the two primary species, *Lactobacillus acidophilus* and *Bifidobacterium bifidum*, along with some of the other species including *Lactobacillus rhamnosus, Lactobacillus casei, Lactobacillus plantarum, Bifidobacteria breve* and *Bifidobacterium longum*.

Dosage: 2 capsules daily between meals.

Other Nutrients

Iron, folate (folic acid), iodine, vitamins B1, B2, B3, B6, B12, E and K, phosphorous, copper, selenium and zinc all play important parts in supporting a healthy pregnancy. If you're taking a quality prenatal vitamin/mineral and maintaining a healthy diet, you probably won't become deficient in any of these particular nutrients. But should a blood test indicate that you are low in one or more of them, your health-care practitioner may recommend that you take additional amounts in the form of a supplement.

Testing for Vitamin/Mineral Deficiencies

A standard blood chemistry panel usually includes serum calcium, phosphorous, sodium, potassium and iron. If your overall health is excellent and there are no other complications, this test may be enough to monitor your nutritional status before and during pregnancy. However, if you have other problems, symptoms or concerns, further testing may be warranted to evaluate the blood levels of all the other vitamins, minerals, fatty acids and amino acids. In this situation, you may want to request a full nutritional profile from your primary physician.

SpectraCell Lab (www.spectracell.com) and MetaMetrix Lab (www.metametrix.com) are two labs in the U.S. that offer specialized test panels for the full range of vitamins, minerals, amino acids and fatty acids.

EXERCISE

Keep the mind still and the body moving.

Many women shy away from any kind of physical exercise during pregnancy because they fear that the baby may suffer damage. In truth, there is no evidence that carefully selected exercise has any negative effect on the unborn baby. On the contrary, pregnant women who regularly exercise at or above 50 percent of their preconception exercise levels have been shown to enjoy the following benefits:

- better immune function and blood pressure[30]

- less discomfort during the third trimester[31]

- shorter labor and delivery times[32]

- lower levels of fetal stress during the birth process[33]

- improved mood[34]

- improved post-partum mood[34]

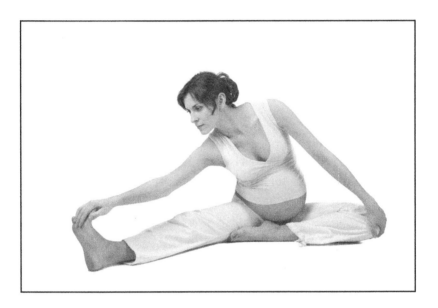

Studies suggest that regular, low-impact aerobic exercise, including walking, stationary cycling, yoga, swimming, and Pilates, are all beneficial and can help ease the mother's physical and mental stress during pregnancy.[35]

A moderate amount of exercise is considered to be the most beneficial, with studies indicating that exercising too much or too little can raise the risk of bearing a low-birth-weight baby. Researchers found that women who exercised strenuously five or more times a week had four times the risk of having a low-birth-weight baby. Women who exercised less than three times a week were twice as likely to have a low-birth-weight baby. *Pregnant women who exercised three or four times each week were found to have the best chance of having a healthy weight baby.*

Some exercises should be completely avoided due to the risk of abdominal injury and strain. They include high-impact aerobics, jogging, skating, skiing (snow and water), scuba diving, weight lifting and horseback riding.

Exercises can also focus on strengthening the muscles of the abdominal wall, pelvis and back to facilitate better support and posture during the second and third trimesters. This will also help make the delivery process easier for the mother. Specific exercises that target these muscle groups include the Kegel and Tailor movements.[36]

HOME ENVIRONMENT

As noted in Chapter 3, our exposure to environmental pollutants and toxins is extreme in this day and age. During pregnancy, you and your baby are most susceptible to the detrimental effects of the chemicals and metals found in a vast array of common household items, including plastics, fabrics, detergents, household cleaners, carpets and furniture, just to name a few.[37] Fortunately, you do have control over your home environment, so you can do a lot to limit your exposure to these toxins in your own home.

Typically, the air quality is four times worse inside a house than it is outside, due to the fact that there is much less ventilation and circulation indoors.[38] You can correct this by purchasing and using a HEPA air filter. HEPA (which stands for high efficiency particulate air) filters can remove at least 99.97 percent of airborne particles 0.3 micrometers in diameter. There are many models and sizes available to suit whatever your home requirements may be.[39,40] (Austin Air is one brand with a very good reputation.)

Below are some other essential ways to improve the quality of your home environment:

- Purify your water supply with high-quality 3-5-stage filtering equipment.

- Use eco-friendly and organic products in your home (biologically safe soaps, detergents, laundry powders and household cleaners).

- Use eco-friendly and organic products on yourself (biologically safe shampoos, toothpaste, creams, cleansers and deodorants).

- Wherever possible, utilize non-toxic paints, furniture, carpets, flooring and cabinets.

(See Chapter 3: Environmental Problems and Solutions for a complete discussion of environmental toxins and how to limit your exposure to them.)

OSTEOPATHY

As your baby grows, and begins to take up more space within you, your internal organs will be moved around, additional body weight will accumulate, your center of gravity will shift, and your posture and sleeping positions will change. These are major structural changes and the reasons that many expectant mothers suffer from pain that settles in the back, neck and other muscular and joint discomfort or pain.

Receiving osteopathic manipulative treatment (OMT) throughout pregnancy is an excellent way to support your musculoskeletal health. A well-trained osteopathic physician can utilize the most sophisticated methods and gentle techniques for keeping your body flexible and open to the many physical changes associated with pregnancy. Osteopathy can

• assist your body in adapting to the physical and structural changes of pregnancy

• support the function of the nervous, circulatory, lymphatic and immune systems

• prepare your pelvis and uterus for labor and delivery

• assist in recovery after the birth

A recent study found that women who received osteopathic care throughout pregnancy had much lower rates of Cesarean section delivery, pre-term delivery, umbilical cord prolapse (a condition in which the umbilical cord precedes the baby, cutting off the oxygen and blood supply) and meconium-stained amniotic fluid (stool in the amniotic fluid), compared to women who did not receive this treatment.[41, 42]

Osteopathy offers benefits for your body, emotions and mind. Find an osteopathic doctor (D.O) whose primary focus and specialty is working as a real and traditional osteopath with OMT.

HOMEOPATHY

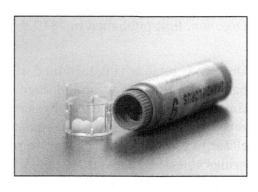

This form of medicine has been in use around the world for over 200 years. Despite this long history and the outstanding results experienced by so many physicians and patients, homeopathy is still misunderstood by many in the pharmaceutical medical community.

There are approximately 2,000 remedies in the homeopathic medicinal repertoire. Each remedy has been extensively tested and observed and a very detailed portrait of all the characteristic physical, emotional and mental signs and symptoms, and life patterns that each remedy addresses has been compiled.

The task of the well-trained Hahnemanian homeopathic physician is to listen to you, your complaints and concerns and observe you and your symptoms. A good homeopath listens carefully to everything you say and notices what you don't say, and observes everything about you, including things that you want to show and things that you don't want to show. The next step is to select the one, single precise remedy that matches your particular signs, symptoms and characteristics. When homeopathy is approached in this manner, the one "constitutional" remedy that is prescribed can touch and heal the deepest part of who you are—your spirit and soul.

Homeopathy is spiritual medicine. It differs from every other form of medicine by virtue of where and how it heals. It is the medicine of the soul. This is the original manner, method and purpose of homeopathy as it was developed by its founder, Samuel Hahnemann, M.D., and meticulously detailed in his treatise, *The Organon*, first published in 1810.[43]

Once your remedy is determined, it can be taken on an ongoing basis, with the potency and dosage adjusted at the appropriate times by your homeopathic physician. As you take a constitutional remedy, it begins to move the innermost parts of who you are closer to your own truth, closer to your own authenticity, which brings you closer to your true destiny. As this process takes place, any emotional and mental aspects that have been out of balance and compromising your life begin to self-correct. As these changes take place, associated physical symptoms, ailments or diseases begin to clear up and move away from you. This is healing from the inside out. Healing deep from within manifests into external reality as you experience greater enjoyment and health in your daily life.

Working with a well-qualified homeopathic physician throughout your pregnancy can be of tremendous benefit to you and your newborn baby, by

- keeping you physically healthy and comfortable during your pregnancy.

- decreasing the likelihood that any negative family genetic predispositions will be passed on to your baby.

- improving your physical, emotional, and mental foundation for after the birth.

ACUPUNCTURE

Acupuncture has a long and well-documented history of preparing mothers-to-be for the birth process and facilitating an easier labor.[44] In a recent study conducted by the New Zealand Midwives Association, it was found that women who received ongoing acupuncture treatments for 3-4 months prior to birth and delivery consistently experienced more efficient labor, with a reduction in the length of labor and amount of medical intervention required. Specifically, the study found decreases of 35 percent in the number of inductions, 35 percent in the epidural rate and 32 percent in emergency cesarean delivery, plus an increase of 9 percent in normal vaginal births.[45, 46]

One acupuncture treatment weekly during the last trimester

of pregnancy is recommended. (Please note: if you are taking a homeopathic constitutional remedy, acupuncture is *not* recommended. You don't need to do both.)

PRE-BIRTH HERBAL, NUTRITIONAL AND HOMEOPATHIC REMEDIES

Certain herbal, nutritional and homeopathic remedies have been shown to be helpful and effective in supporting labor and the birth process when taken during pregnancy. The most important and effective are

Herbal

Raspberry Leaf Tea

Tea made from the raspberry leaf has a long history of use in herbal medicine as a uterine tonic and cervical conditioner. In a study conducted by the Australian Midwives Association, it was shown that women who drank this tea throughout their pregnancy, and in particular during the last 3-4 weeks prior to delivery, experienced shorter and easier labor with fewer forceps deliveries.[47] It is recommended that 1-3 cups be taken daily during the 3-4 weeks prior to the expected birth date.

Nutritional

Evening Primrose Oil

Evening primrose oil (an omega-6 fatty acid) can help soften and "ripen" the uterus and cervix prior to delivery, due to the effects of regulating prostaglandins within the body. Prostaglandins are responsible for regulating the degree of inflammatory response and flexibility in many tissues of the body, including the uterus and cervix. Take one 500 mg capsule 3 times daily with meals for 3-4 weeks prior to the expected birth date.[48]

Homeopathic

Caulophyllum

Caulophyllum is the primary homeopathic remedy to consider for assisting the uterus and cervix in delivery. If everything in your pregnancy is progressing well, help your body prepare for the birth by taking caulophyllum 12c, one pellet twice daily for the 2 weeks prior to the expected birth date.[49] If you are experiencing any complications during your pregnancy, consult with a well-qualified homeopathic practitioner before taking this remedy.

All of the above supplements and remedies can be taken in addition to the recommended supplements that you have been taking throughout your pregnancy.

THE BABY ARRIVES

Birth is the second major transition for a person entering into this world. During the first transition, the baby's soul enters the mother's womb where there is protection, warmth and nourishment. Outside the womb, there are new people, noises and lights, a mass of swirling energy and impressions. This is your baby's experience of life in this world. The birth should always be as warm, welcoming and authentic as possible, for first impressions have a lasting impact, consciously and unconsciously. The environment, surroundings, obstetrician, midwife, doula and any medical interventions administered at birth are all very personal choices that only the mother and father can make. Consider carefully what will be most comfortable for you and best for your baby.

In addition to these natural challenges, the hospital may want to give your newborn baby a shocking and immune-altering injection of hepatitis B vaccine in the first few hours following his or her birth.[50] I have discussed the details regarding children's vaccinations, and the long-lived controversy among medical professionals, in Chapter 5. However, at this stage, it is important to point out how dramatic and potentially dangerous it is for newborns to be injected with genetic material and toxic chemicals in the first hours of their outside life. It will always be a personal decision for the parents whether to vaccinate your infant or not, but I would always recommend to both parents and for your newborn baby's sake to never allow your baby to receive this hepatitis B injection at birth. Delay the decision until you have a chance to be fully informed and educated and at the very least, given time for your baby to arrive and settle in.

Osteopathy

During labor and birth, your baby's head and body will undergo major compression while moving down the birth canal. It is not unusual during this birth "trauma" for the baby's head to become compressed, resulting in a somewhat misshapen head. A skull that stays compressed after birth may contribute to colic, restlessness, sleeplessness, developmental disorders or hyperactivity.[51, 52] The benefits of providing your baby with osteopathic treatment after the birth to assist in decompressing the cranial plates are supported by the medical literature. Providing mother with osteopathic treatment after delivery is also highly recommended, as it can help the body realign and readjust after undergoing the dramatic changes and structural stresses of nine months of pregnancy and the delivery process.

Homeopathy

Following the birth, you may also want to utilize certain homeopathic remedies to help you recover from any bruising, tearing or discomfort. They include:

- *Arnica 30 c* – for any bruising, soreness, swelling and discomfort following delivery.

- *Calendula 30c* – for any tearing and/or associated bleeding.

- *Caulophyllum 30 c* – for overall muscular weakness, exhaustion and nervousness after delivery.

- *Cimicifuga 30 c* – for after-pains that involve violent spasms and aches in the pelvic area. These pains may be associated with fear and dejection.

- *Pulsatilla 30 c* – for after-pains, when there is weepiness, much need for emotional support, company and closeness.

- *Sepia 30 c* – for pains that are felt as a weight or bearing down, as if your uterus would fall out, and/or if feeling emotionally irritable or edgy, with a desire to be by yourself.

- *China 30 c* – for pains or weakness associated with loss of blood or other bodily fluids leading to dehydration, faintness, fatigue and extreme sensitivity to all environmental stimuli.

These homeopathic remedies can be used safely and effectively after birth and while you are breastfeeding your baby.[53] Ideally, you should consult with your homeopath to select the most appropriate remedy. Typically in this situation, the dosage would be one pellet three times daily until all symptoms are improved.

WELCOME, BABY!

When your baby re-enters this world through you and with you, the deepest level at which you, the mother, can welcome and assure the arrival is by acknowledging and embracing his or her soul. This goes beyond words, beyond the intellect, beyond the mind. It goes to the place where there is no time, no words, but everything exists. It goes to the place where hearts connect, touch and embrace silently and completely.

Chapter 8

Optimal Health: Breastfeeding and Infant's Diet

Your newborn baby has very simple, pure needs: nourishment, warmth, protection and love. Nature displays her intelligence by knowing that breastfeeding your baby satisfies all of these needs simultaneously and in the most tangible way.

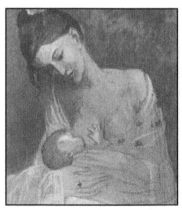

Everyone agrees that breastfeeding is the ideal way to feed an infant throughout the first year. How long to continue doing so is a very personal decision. Most would agree that if a mother can continue breastfeeding for at least a year, the baby will get an excellent start in life.

MOTHER'S DIET WHILE BREASTFEEDING

As with your diet during pregnancy, you are still eating for both you and your baby while you are nursing. Protein remains of utmost importance, along with the right balance of carbohydrates (vegetables, fruit, grains such as rice, pasta, noodles and bread), and fats and oils (olive oil, flaxseed oil, butter, coconut oil).

Key Guidelines

- Eat well-balanced meals that contain protein, vegetables, grains and good fats and oils (olive oil, flaxseed oil, butter) at each meal. Include plenty of fresh fruits.

- Drink at least six 8-ounce glasses of pure, clean water daily.

- Consume at least 1,000 mg of calcium daily. This can be accomplished with a healthy diet. Dairy products (milk, yogurt, cheese and kefir) are good sources of calcium along with broccoli, collard greens, kale, mustard greens, turnip greens, bok choy, canned salmon, sardines, almonds and brazil nuts. If you do not tolerate or eat many dairy products, you may consider supplementing your diet with a calcium/magnesium supplement (500 mg 1-2 times daily with food).

- Be careful with the consumption of fish. Avoid shark, swordfish and king mackerel at all times due to their high mercury content. Limit tuna to no more than 12 ounces per week, also due to mercury content. Avoid shellfish, and bottom dwelling fish such as catfish, eel, sole, and flounder due to their high degree of bacterial, viral and fecal contamination.

- Avoid coffee. Studies show that coffee overload can cause the same symptoms in your baby as it does in you: nervousness, edginess, irritability and insomnia.

- Avoid alcohol. All forms of alcohol can affect the nervous system and impede the brain development of a young baby.

- Be careful with strong-flavored and spicy foods, which can easily irritate and aggravate your baby's digestive and nervous system.

- Check your iron levels with a blood test; iron is one of the most important minerals for your baby's growth at this age and also one of the most common deficiencies found in nursing mothers. This can be easily checked with blood work from your doctor.

Follow the Blood Type Diet

This diet is good for you at any time, and will be especially helpful during nursing. If you and your baby share the same blood type, this makes it very easy. If your baby's blood type is different than yours, review both blood type food lists to determine the beneficial foods that you have in common and stick to those. Eating for both you and your baby's blood type will benefit you both and be especially helpful and important if your baby has difficulties such as excess gas, colic, irregular bowel movements, or diet-related skin rashes.

Take Supplements

The supplements recommended during breastfeeding are the same as those needed during the prenatal period. They include

- *Prenatal vitamin/mineral* – Continue taking a quality prenatal vitamin/mineral to ensure that you and your baby are receiving all of the essential vitamins and minerals required for growth, development and maintenance.

  Dosage: Follow recommendation on the product label.

- *Cod liver oil* — Sixty percent of the brain is made up of fats and oils, and 60 percent of these fats and oils consist of one particular fatty acid called docosahexaenoic acid (DHA).[1] Cod liver oil contains high levels of naturally occurring DHA, which is essential for supporting and nourishing your baby's brain development. A study in the *Journal of Pediatrics* published in 2003, demonstrated that women who supplemented their diets with cod liver oil during pregnancy and while breastfeeding increased their child's intelligence by an average of 4.1 IQ points by the age of 4 years.[2, 3] Imagine increasing your child's intelligence simply by adding cod liver oil to your diet. In addition, DHA and the omega-3 oils can help regulate your hormones, reduce the chance of postpartum depression and improve your mood.

Dosage: 1 tablespoon or three 1,000 mg capsules of cod liver oil daily with meals. (Make sure they are certified free of mercury, PCBs and dioxins.)

- *Probiotics* - Take 2 capsules daily of a probiotic that contains both the *Acidophilus* and *Bifidobacteria* species (*Lactobacillus acidophilus, Bifidobacterium bifidum,* along with other species such as *Lactobacillus rhamnosus, Lactobacillus casei, Lactobacillus plantarum*). A good-quality probiotic will help maintain and support intestinal ecology, integrity and immunity, which is beneficial to the immune and digestive systems of both you and your baby.[4]

Dosage: 1-2 capsules daily between meals.

INFANT'S DIET—FORMULA

If breastfeeding your infant is not an option, or you need to supplement your nursing, you'll want to find the best pediatric formula available for your baby. When choosing a formula, I recommend the following:

- Use an infant formula based on goat's milk or cow's milk.

- Only use a soy-based formula as a last resort, when allergies to goat's milk or cow's milk are proven. (Use soy-based formula only when prescribed and supervised by a health professional.)

- Only use certified organic formulas.

- Choose the formula that best suits your baby's blood type.

Goat's Milk Vs. Cow's Milk

Although we in the Western world think of cow's milk as *the* drink for children, the reality is that most of the world's children grow up on goat's milk. Some 70 percent of children worldwide grow up drinking goat's milk. When we compare the two, we see that goat's milk makes far more sense for the majority of children. Consider the following:

- *Goat's milk is less allergenic*

  Milk allergies are reactions to a protein allergen known as Alpha s1 Casein, which is found in high levels in cow's milk. The levels of Alpha s1 Casein in goat's milk are about 85 percent less than cow's milk, making it a far less allergenic food.

- *Goat's milk is naturally homogenized*

  Goat's milk has smaller fat globules and does not contain agglutinin, a compound found in cow's milk that causes the milk to separate into two layers—cream and the skim milk. With smaller fat globules and no agglutinin, the goat's milk stays naturally homogenized (mixed), making it easier to digest.

- *Goat's milk is easier to digest*

When goat's milk proteins denature (clump together) in the stomach, they form a much softer bolus (curd) than the bolus formed by cow's milk. This allows the body to digest the protein more easily and completely. In addition, goat's milk contains higher levels of medium-chain fatty acids than cow's milk, which also make it far easier to digest.

- *Goat's milk rarely causes lactose intolerance*

  Goat's milk contains less lactose than cow's milk and therefore is easier to digest for those suffering from lactose intolerance. Although goat's milk contains only about 10 percent less lactose than cow's milk, it has been noted that the lactose intolerance problems seen with cow's milk are often nonexistent with goat's milk. This may be due to the overall easier digestibility of goat's milk.

- *Goat's milk contains extra vitamins and fatty acids*

  Compared to cow's milk, goat's milk contains higher amounts of vitamin A, vitamin B6, niacin, potassium and the essential fatty acids, linoleic acid and arachidonic acid.

- *Goat's milk is an alkaline food*

  The higher potassium content of goat's milk creates an alkaline effect within the body, instead of the acidifying reaction created by cow's milk. Maintaining an alkaline pH environment has significant health benefits by improving the body's cellular ability to absorb nutrients and efficiently remove waste.

- *Goat's milk was designed for a similar-size baby*

  Cow's milk is designed to feed a 100-pound calf, which will eventually develop into a 1,000-pound cow. Goat's milk, on the other hand, is designed to feed a 7-10-pound kid, which will eventually develop into an adult that weighs 120-200 pounds. From this we can see that goat's milk and human milk are both designed to feed a 7-10-pound infant, who will then grow to a similar size and weight as an adult.

- *Goat's milk contains more calcium* than cow's milk, and provides comparable amounts of all the other vitamins and minerals except for folic acid and vitamin B12. These two vitamins can be easily added to goat's milk if needed.

Stay Away from Soy Formula, if Possible

Soy naturally contains phytoestrogens, plant-based compounds that act like a mild form of estrogen in the body. Because they act like hormones in the body, phytoestrogens may contribute to thyroid problems in babies who have a genetic predisposition towards them.[5] Phytoestrogens may also affect other aspects of the developing hormonal system in babies and young children, particularly in boys. For example, increased estrogen levels may cause boys to acquire more feminine attributes and interfere with proper development of the genitalia.[6, 7]

While soy and soy products can be beneficial for adults with A and AB blood types, and okay for adults with blood types B and O, they are not recommended for babies and infants due to the vulnerability and sensitivity of their delicate and developing hormonal systems. Thus, I suggest that you refrain from giving soy formula to your baby, unless there are special circumstances such as lactose intolerance or a proven cow's milk protein intolerance, and there is no other alternative.

The New Zealand Ministry of Health summed up the situation very well in its guidelines for use of soy-based formula, with these recommendations formulated after an extensive review of the literature on the subject:

"Soy formula should only be used under the direction of a health professional for specific medical indications, such as a proven cow's milk protein intolerance or allergy, or lactose intolerance. Health professionals undertaking dietary treatment of these conditions should first consider the use of alternative non-soy-based infant formulas, which are available [e.g., goat milk formulas].... Clinicians who are treating children with a soy-based infant formula should be aware of the potential interaction between soy infant formula and thyroid function and should consider ongoing assessment of thyroid function."[8]

Formulas for Special Needs

For babies with digestive problems such as colic, gassiness, constipation, diarrhea, or related symptoms such as skin rashes, eczema, or recurrent ear infections, consider trying a formula that contains milk protein that has been instantized (partially broken down into a smaller size making it easier to digest, assimilate and metabolize). Nestle's "Good Start" is the primary formula of this kind in the U.S.

For highly allergic babies or those with severe digestive difficulties, there are extensively hydrolyzed, hypoallergenic formulas containing milk proteins that are broken down to an even smaller size than those found in the instantized formulas. The primary formulas in this category are Nutramigen, Pregestamil and Alimentum. Generally, these specialty formulas will be recommended and prescribed by a pediatrician.

Use a Certified Organic Formula Only

A newborn baby should ideally *only* be given an organic formula, to eliminate exposure to chemical additives, pesticides, herbicides, hormones or antibiotics. Make sure the formula is *certified* organic. Surprisingly, this will rule out the majority of infant formulas on the market today.

In the U.S. there are three original brands of organic formulas: Baby's Only, Earth's Best and UltraBright Beginnings. All are respectable and available in both cow's milk and soy-based formulas.

In the U.S., mass market brands like Similac and Parents Choicehave recently introduced organic versions of their formulas. This is significant, as it shows that these manufacturers, who control 95 percent of the infant formula market, have finally realized that parents are seeking organic foods for their children beginning at birth, and will not accept formulas that contain chemicals, pesticides, hormones or antibiotics.

Other Organic Formulas Available Worldwide

Cow's Milk Formula

In England, Europe and New Zealand the organic cow's milk formula that is available is Babynat.

Goat's Milk Formula

The primary brand of organic goat's milk formula in Europe is Holle , which is also available around the world via the Internet.

In New Zealand, the Dairy Goat Cooperative produces its own goat's milk formula. In Australia, Bellamy's Organic infant formula is available in cow's milk, goat's milk or soy-based formulas.

Determining Formula Base by Baby's Blood Type

One way of selecting a formula base—cow's milk, goat's milk or soy milk—involves determining the kind that best suits your baby's blood type. The recomended types of formula for each blood type are as follows:

Blood Type O
First Choice – Organic goat's milk formula

Second Choice – Organic cow's milk formula (if above is not possible)

Third Choice – Soy formula (if allergy to both goat and cow milk is proven through allergy testing)

Blood Type A
First Choice – Organic goat's milk formula

Second Choice – Organic cow's milk formula (if above is not possible)

Third Choice – Soy formula (if allergy to both goat and cow milk is proven)

Blood Type B
First Choice — Organic cow's milk formula

Second Choice – Organic goat's milk formula

Third Choice — Soy formula (if allergy to both goat and cow milk is proven)

Blood Type AB

First Choice – Organic goat's milk formula

Second Choice – Organic cow's milk formula

Third Choice – Soy formula (if allergy to both goat and cow milk is proven)

	Units	Human	Cow	Goat	Soy
Calories	kcal	160	160	167	140
Protein	g	1	3.22	3.56	6.74
Fat	g	4	3.25	4.14	4.67
Carbohydrate	g	6.9	4.52	4.45	4.43
Fiber	g	0	0	0	1.3
Calcium	mg	34	113	134	38
Magnesium	mg	3	10	14	25
Sodium	mg	23	40	50	55
Potassium	mg	51	143	204	124
Iron	mg	0.03	0.03	0.05	1.1
Zinc	mg	0.17	0.4	0.3	0.44
Selenium	mg	1.8	3.7	1.4	4.8
Manganese	mg	0.03	0.03	0.02	0.22
Vitamin A	mg	32	102	198	31
Vitamin C	mg	5	0	1.3	0
Vitamin D	mg	0.3	40	12	16
Vitamin E	mg	0.3	0.06	0.07	1.35
Vitamin B1	mg	0.01	0.04	0.05	0.06
Vitamin B2	mg	0.04	0.18	0.14	0.05
Vitamin B5	mg	0.22	0.36	0.31	0.31
Vitamin B6	mg	0.01	0.04	0.05	0.1
Vitamin B12	mg	0.05	0.44	0.07	1.22
Vitamin K	mcg	0.3	0.2	0.3	3
Folate	mcg	5	5	1	16

Source: USDA Nutrient Data Base
Online at http://www.nal.usda.gov/fnic/foodcomp/search/

Comparison of Nutritional Content of Human, Cow, Goat and Soy Milk

INTRODUCING SOLID FOODS

Ask ten different pediatricians or other medical professionals when to start introducing solid foods to your baby and you'll probably get ten different answers. However, the first and most important thing to keep in mind is that every child is unique and develops at his or her own rate. While there are general guidelines for introducing solid foods, there is no set time, no rule, and no pre-determined age that applies to all children. Instead, the introduction of solid foods is best determined on an individual basis.

It will depend on your baby's development, overall health, constitution and levels of interest in food. It will depend on whether or not there are any symptoms of digestive trouble, allergies or sensitivities such as skin rashes, eczema, recurrent diaper rash, constipation, diarrhea, excess gassiness, fussiness, irritability or disturbed sleep. If any of these are present, the timing of the introduction of solid foods and the foods offered become even more important.

It's very important that you refrain from rushing the introduction of solid foods. Giving solid foods to your baby before their digestive system is ready will dramatically increase the risk of creating food allergies, sensitivities and digestive problems, all of which affect the immune and nervous system. This will make your child more susceptible to a host of other conditions, including rashes, eczema, recurrent ear infections, mood disturbances and sleeping problems.

Uppermost in your mind should be an awareness of nature's wisdom and clues. The teeth, for example, are the biggest clue indicating when your child is ready for solid food. Your baby's tooth development correlates with the development of the digestive system. Thus, when the teeth are ready, the digestive system is also ready. Some children start teething at 5-6 months of age, while others may not start until 9-10 months. That's why you can't pinpoint an exact age for the introduction of solid foods, although most pediatricians recommend that you consider beginning at about 6 months of age.

Signs of Readiness

I suggest you wait until your child is 6 months old, and then look for these indications of readiness for solid foods:

- Presence of teeth

- Baby can sit up and support his or her own head. To eat solid foods an infant needs to have good head and neck control and should be able to sit up.

- Baby shows interest in solid food. Staring at and reaching for your food at the dinner table is sign of readiness.

- Baby's current state of health is good, particularly in relation to the digestive system (e.g., no bloating, gassiness, diarrhea, constipation, or skin rashes).

Let your baby's readiness be the determining factor when timing the introduction of solid foods.

Principles for Introducing Solid Foods

Observing the following principles will ensure that your child and his or her digestive and immune systems receive the best possible start in life:

- Choose from the foods that suit your baby's blood type. (See discussion of the Blood Type Diet in Chapter 1.)

- Always use organic foods.

- Over time, introduce a variety of foods to create a healthy and balanced diet and allowing your baby to experience a range of tastes, textures and nutrients.

As you begin introducing your baby to foods, remember that he or she is forming habits, tendencies and patterns that will remain for a lifetime. Make these experiences healthy and happy ones.

Stage One (6-8 months)

When introducing solid food, go slowly and be patient. Expect that more of it will end up dribbling down your baby's chin than going down his or her throat. But that's okay—swallowing solid food taken from a spoon takes a lot of practice!

Start with Rice Cereal

Rice cereal is typically the very first food introduced to babies, as almost all babies tolerate and digest it well. This is borne out by the Blood Type Diet, which recommends rice for all four blood types as it seems to suit everybody.

At the beginning, mix 1-2 teaspoons of organic brown rice cereal with 4-5 tsp breast milk or formula and offer it once daily. Gradually increase to twice daily.

Then Try Vegetables and Fruits

Once your baby is able to handle rice cereal with no digestive problems, you can begin to introduce vegetables and fruits. Start with the vegetables first, as the sweetness of the fruits may compromise the baby's taste for vegetables. Foods that are commonly introduced first may include

- Vegetables: sweet potatoes, squash, carrots, green beans and peas

- Fruits: apples, pears, bananas and avocados

These foods have been found over time to be appealing and easily digested. However, be sure to introduce one food at a time and wait at least one week before introducing another food so you can watch for and note any reactions, especially the following:

- Digestive distress: bloating, excessive gas, diarrhea, irritability

- Skin problems: itching, swelling, hives or rashes

- Respiratory distress: congestion, mucus, coughing or wheezing

- Mood disturbances: irritability, crying, disturbed sleep

If any of these symptoms begin to appear, look to the most recent food that you offered. If you are introducing one food at a time and allowing a week in between, the culprit should be obvious. You may also want to re-evaluate all of the foods your baby is eating. Make sure each food suits your baby's blood type. Also be certain that they are completely organic to rule out the possibility that added chemicals may be causing the reaction.

If symptoms continue, consult with a homeopathic, naturopathic or osteopathic physician.

Stage Two (8-10 months)

After spending a couple of months introducing the foods listed above, if all goes well you can start to introduce other foods as well as food blends. Continue to select foods according to the food list that suits your baby's blood type, and introduce them one at a time.

New Foods to Introduce

The foods that you might consider next include

- Grains: amaranth, buckwheat, millet, quinoa (the gluten-free grains)

- Vegetables: broccoli, zucchini, eggplant, cauliflower, potatoes

- Fruits: peaches, apricots, nectarines, plums, prunes, grapes, dates, figs, cherries, melons

- Protein: chicken, turkey

Stage Three (10-12 months)

Meats, poultry and fish can be added toward the end of the first year when the digestive system and kidneys are ready to metabolize the protein. At this stage, you may also introduce

- Grains: rice crackers, rice pasta (avoid all wheat products and the other grains that contain gluten:- barley, bulgur, rye, spelt, kamut, couscous, matzo, semolina. Oats do not contain gluten; however, because they are always processed in the same mills, processing plants and grain elevators as wheat, barley and rye, this results in enough contamination of oats with these other grains that they can often trigger the same reaction.)

- <u>Vegetables:</u> asparagus, spinach, beets

- <u>Fruits:</u> blueberries, cantaloupe, kiwi, mango, papaya

- <u>Protein:</u> beans, legumes, lentils, lean ground beef, lamb, fish

Highest allergy foods

The foods that cause allergic reactions most often, according to the U.S. FDA[9],are

- Wheat

- Cow's milk

- Soy products

- Crustacean shellfish

- Eggs

- Peanuts

- Tree nuts

- Fish

In addition, foods that are most likely to cause reactions in babies during the first 1-2 years include

- Citrus fruits

- Strawberries

- Chocolate

It is recommended that you avoid giving your child citrus fruits, strawberries and chocolate during the first year. After your child's first birthday, you can evaluate the suitability of any of these foods based on his or her blood type.

FOOD FOR THOUGHT

During the first year of life, a baby typically triples his or her birth weight, approaching the quadruple mark by the end of the second year. This huge amount of proportional growth is supported by breast milk (or formula) during the first six months or so, then breast milk (or formula) in conjunction with solid foods for the next six months, and solid foods during the second year.

Researchers have found that a child's earliest eating habits and food choices will determine his or her future food choices, weight and health. An eight-year study of 70 mother/baby pairs performed at the University of Tennessee and published in 2002, confirmed that food preferences are established early: 8-year-olds usually like the same foods they did when they were 4, and their preferences are often formed as early as age 2.[10]

Unfortunately, these preferences are often of the unhealthy kind. In 2002, the U.S. Government "Feeding Infants and Toddlers Study" (FITS) found that 25 percent of 9-11-month-olds were not even consuming one helping of vegetables a day. Potatoes were the most commonly consumed vegetable at 9 months of age, and 13 percent of 12-month-olds ate French fries every day—becoming the number one vegetable consumed by U.S. toddlers. By age 2, 1 in 5 babies were eating candy every day.[11]

In light of the terrible dietary habits that have developed in recent years, it's not surprising that during the past 15 years, the U.S., Europe and all developed Westernized countries have experienced an epidemic of childhood obesity and the associated conditions of hypertension, elevated cholesterol and type 2 diabetes in children. The number of children suffering from these disorders is expected to increase exponentially in the near future.[12, 13] The current U.S National Health and Nutrition Examination Survey found that 14 percent of 2-5-year-olds are overweight or obese, more than twice the number seen in the mid-1970s, and a 35 percent increase in the past four years alone. Another 26 percent of 2-5-year-olds are at risk of developing these conditions.[14, 15] Obesity and type 2 diabetes are inextricably linked to the poor dietary habits of high-calorie, low-nutrient foods in infancy and childhood.

A recent study conducted by University College London and published in the *Journal of Psychiatry* (Nov. 2009) found that a diet heavy in processed and fatty foods also increases the risk of depression. The participants who mainly ate fried food, processed meat, high-fat dairy products and sweetened desserts had a 58 percent higher incidence of depression.

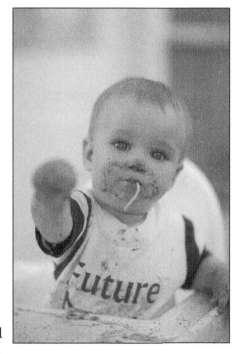

There is no mystery or controversy. A healthy diet is the cornerstone for a long and healthy life. Encouraging and forming healthy eating habits in childhood is the beginning of that journey.

Never forget that the foods you provide and the eating habits you help establish in infancy will affect your child, positively or negatively, for a lifetime.

Diet is king and exercise is queen.
                    —*Jack LaLanne, "the godfather of fitness," at 95*

Chapter 9

Optimal Health: Toddlerhood into Childhood—Putting it all Together

During your baby's first year, he or she has traveled from the world of the souls to your womb, then out into this world to nurse, teethe, eat solid food, crawl, walk and talk. Your focus should be to support, nourish and encourage good health, while guarding against anything that can interfere with the full physical, emotional, mental and spiritual development of your child.

The primary physical factors that influence your child's health include

- food and diet

- movement and exercise

- contact with environmental toxins

- exposure to antibiotics and vaccinations

Vaccinations are discussed extensively in Chapter 5 and Appendix

II. Medical treatments and the best methods for addressing any ailments that may arise are covered in Appendix I. In this chapter we will focus on food, diet, supplementation, exercise and preventative medical care.

FOOD AND DIET FOR THE TODDLER

By the age of one year, most children are ready to be introduced to the whole spectrum of food choices. The exception is the infant with an especially sensitive digestive system and/or food allergies (conditions that are often seen together), which may warrant a delay in introducing new foods or omitting certain foods altogether. (*See* Chapter 2.)

Now is the time to establish the best dietary choices and habits for your child. The dietary habits and patterns created during infancy and early childhood will influence the food choices your child will make for the rest of his or her life, so this is a vitally important task.

The primary principles for a healthy diet, as detailed in previous chapters, remain the same:

- **Provide clean, organic foods**

- **Provide the foods that best suit your child's blood type**

- **Avoid non-kosher foods**

- **Provide clean, pure water**

- **At food and meal times, there should be time to relax and enjoy each other, and the food. Relax and enjoy your meals and your child will, too.**

The following conclusions were drawn from one of the most extensive, useful and detailed studies of its kind, conducted at the University of Minnesota in the U.S.:

- What the parents eat is the primary influencing factor in shaping what children eat, from 2 years of age through the teens.

- Try 10 times—that is the average number of times that an infant needs to try a new food before liking it, so keep offering healthful food choices, even if your child seems uninterested at first. Familiarity will increase his or her desire and intake.

- Resist the temptation to bargain, as in "Eat your vegetables and you can have dessert." This only creates a power struggle over food. Choose when to eat and what to provide, and then your child can choose what to consume from what you have offered.[1]

The study, which included 36,000 Minnesota teens, also showed the direct correlation between academic performance and a healthy diet. Teens who earned the highest grades were the ones who had a history of consuming a more nutritious diet, including more fruits and vegetables.[2]

Proportions and a Balanced Diet

Once you are obtaining and giving your child fresh, clean, organic and kosher foods that suit his or her particular blood type, the final aspect to a completely healthy diet is the right proportion and balance of foods, namely, the right proportion of proteins, carbohydrates fats and oils to be served at each meal.

By balancing the amount and intake of proteins, carbohydrates, fats and oils, you create a balanced metabolism, which then allows the smooth, steady conversion and absorption of nutrients and glucose.

You do not have to count calories and measure serving sizes to have a healthy meal. A balanced diet is not difficult to do but includes a few important guidelines and principles. The following paragraphs provide all you need to know and understand to achieve a balanced diet.

Glycemic Index

This is a method that ranks foods (primarily carbohydrate foods) according to their impact on blood sugar. The faster the food is digested and absorbed in the small intestine, the faster and higher the blood sugar will rise and the higher the glycemic index (GI) rating of that food is.

As an example, pure glucose can be absorbed directly into the bloodstream, and on a scale of zero to 100, has a GI rating of 100. Table sugar (sucrose) has a GI rating of 68. White bread, another carbohydrate, has a GI rating of 70. Brown rice has a GI of 50, peas are at 22, carrots are at 16 and onions at 10.[3]

All of the carbohydrate foods (grains, pasta, breads, beans, vegetables and fruit) can be rated as either low-GI (1-30) carbohydrates (vegetables, beans, some fruits), or as medium-to-high GI (35-100) carbohydrates (bread, potato, pasta, rice, desserts). Foods that do not contain carbohydrates, such as protein foods and fats, do not have a direct effect on blood sugar, so their GI rating is zero.

Balancing each meal with the right proportion of proteins, low glycemic carbohydrates along with the good fats and oils is the key to a healthy diet, a healthy child and a long, healthy life at the correct weight.

The following chart shows a list of the most common carbohydrate foods with their glycemic index rating.

Glycemic Index for Various Foods			
Food	GI Index	Food - continued	GI Index
Glucose	100	Pumpernickel Bread	50
Boiled, peeled potato	88	Whole Wheat Bread	49
Baked potato	85	Fresh Peas	48
Cornflakes	81	Oat Bran Breads	47
Boiled, unpeeled potatoes	80	Grapes	46
White Flour	75	Orange Juice	46
Chips/French Fies	75	Oranges	42
Watermelon	72	Fresh Apple Juice	40
Cornflour	70	Spaghetti (al dente)	39
White Bread	70	Apples	38
Sugar (scurose)	68	Pears	38
Cantalope Melon	65	Vanilla Ice cream	37
Mars Bar	65	Whole Wheat Spaghetti	37
Raisins	64	Low-fat Yogurt	33

Glycemic Index for Various Foods			
Food	GI Index	Food - continued	GI Index
Sweet Potato	61	Butter Beans	32
Basmati Rice	58	Dried Apricots	31
Boiled Carrots	58	Green Beans	29
Cola	58	Kidney Beans	28
Long-grain White Rice	56	Chickpeas, Boiled	28
Frosted Cornflakes	55	Whole Milk	27
Honey	55	Red Lentils	26
Digestive Biscuits	55	Grapefruit	25
Brown Rice	55	Dark Chocolate (70%)	22
Oat Bran	55	Cherries	22
Potato chips	54	Fructose	19
Peaches	53	Raw Carrots	16
Kiwi Fruit	53	Peanuts	14
Sweetcorn	53	Onion	10
Banana	52	Garlic	10

Now we go to the final step of putting it all together by combining the right proportions of proteins to carbohydrates to fats and oils for each meal.

Imagine a plate and divide it into thirds. Imagine one-third of the plate contains the protein (meats, poultry, fish, eggs, cheese). Another third of the plate contains the low-GI carbohydrate foods (vegetables, legumes, beans). The final third of the plate contains the medium-to-high GI carbohydrate foods (rice, pasta, potato). Now, add in the use of the healthy omega-3 oils such as olive oil, flaxseed oil, along with the nuts and seeds that suit your child's blood type, and you are providing all the right foods in the right proportions.

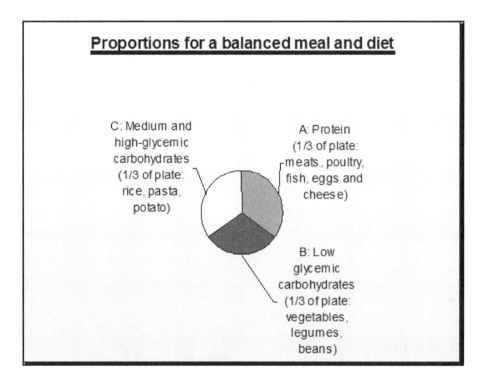

Each meal should also contain healthy omega 3 oils, such as olive and flaxseed oil.

Nutritional Supplementation

For the majority of toddlers and children growing up in today's world, the addition of quality nutritional supplements to their diet will be of great benefit. As mentioned in previous chapters, the right nutritional supplements can ensure your child is receiving all of the essential vitamins, minerals and essential fatty acids that he or she requires to grow and develop properly. In addition, the antioxidant vitamins and minerals can provide your child the extra protection needed these days to neutralize exposure to environmental pollutants and toxins. The correct supplementation program should also provide immune support to keep your child's immune and defense system at full strength and ready for any challenge that he or she may encounter.

Generally, the best time to introduce nutritional supplements will be in your child's first year, after he or she has started eating solid foods, and after you have stopped nursing.

Key Supplements:

- multivitamin/mineral

- cod liver oil

- vitamin C

- probiotics

Multivitamin/mineral

A quality multivitamin/mineral should contain all 14 of the essential vitamins and at least 8 of the primary minerals (calcium, magnesium, potassium, zinc, selenium, manganese, chromium, iodine). Studies have repeatedly shown that children who are supplemented with a good multivitamin/mineral demonstrate improved mental development. They also show children performing significantly better in reading speed, learning capacity, arithmetic examinations and attention scores.[4]

Dosage: Give 5 days per week at the label-recommended dosages for your child's age.

Cod Liver Oil

I have sung the praises of cod liver oil throughout this book and continue here with the recommendation to start supplementing with quality cod liver oil in your baby's first year. Cod liver oil contains the ideal balance of omega-3 fatty acids (DHA and EPA), along with vitamin A (retinol for eye development) and vitamin D (for immune and bone growth).

This is the perfect nutritional supplement for a growing infant, toddler and child. Studies have demonstrated that just supplementing with cod liver oil during pregnancy and while nursing can increase the IQ of a child by up to 5 points by the age of 4 years.[5] Continue to support and encourage your child's brain growth and development with this important supplement.

Dosage: Give 5 days per week at the label-recommended dosages for your child's age.

Vitamin C

This is the superstar vitamin for improving immune function, providing immune protection and protecting your child from all manner of environmental pollutants and toxins. Studies show that when vitamin C is taken on a regular basis, children do not get sick as often or as easily and show a quicker recovery time if they do catch a cold, cough or flu.[6] Vitamin C should always be a part of your child's supplementation.

Dosage: Give 5 days per week at the label-recommended dosages for your child's age.

Probiotics

Lactobacillus acidophilus and *Bifidobacterium bifidum* are the primary probiotic species for children. Along with these two species, additional species that are also very good are *Bifidobacterium longum* and *Bifido bacterium infantis*. These probiotics provide protection against potentially harmful bacteria, yeast, parasites as well as help to digest and metabolize vitamins within the small intestine. In addition, these beneficial bacteria produce lactic acid, a naturally occurring antibacterial substance that provides another layer of immune protection.[7] Providing your child with a good probiotic supplement that contains these species can help to maintain digestive and immune health.

Dosage: Give 2-3 days per week at the label-recommended dosages for your child's age.

Successful Treatment

Luis was 8 years old when I first saw him in the beginning of 2009.

He had a history of recurrent ear infections for which he had been placed on prophylactic antibiotics over the course of six months before having ear tubes placed. He had previously been tested for food allergies and tested positive for wheat and corn, though removing these from his diet had not seemed to make much difference.

He had always been a little anxious and agitated. His teacher reported that it was difficult for him to sit still and focus, and he was always fidgeting, moving and joking around. More recently, he had become angrier and he had shown some bullying behavior. The school principal had recently voiced his concerns about Luis's attention problems and bullying behavior to his mother.

Looking at Luis's history, there were some earlier emotional stresses and traumas that he had been exposed to when his parents separated, and the ongoing antibiotic use over the course of a year had probably stressed his immune and nervous system even more. The result of this was an increase

---

in the degree of his symptoms, where the underlying anxiety and agitation increased to include overt anger and bullying.

His mother took good care with his diet, so we started Luis on his homeopathic constitutional remedy: Hyoscyamus 6 c, once daily, and nutritional supplements to support his digestive and immune system (multivitamin/mineral, probiotics and DHA from cod liver oil).

At his first six-week follow-up visit, his mother told me that she began to see changes after the first two weeks. He was a little calmer, had more self-awareness, noticing when he became agitated, which then allowed him to communicate this and then relax. He had become more responsive to her requests and he had read a whole book for the very first time in his life.

Luis remains on his homeopathic remedy and supplements and continues to do well.

Health Maintenance and Wellness

As we have seen in previous chapters, most regular allopathic pharmaceutical medical care is aimed at "disease care," treating symptoms and illness after they have occurred. True medicine and holistic medical care is aimed at "health care," or preventative care and maintenance that keeps an individual healthy, happy and wise. In Chapter 5, we looked at the main schools of holistic medical care and how you can utilize these methods to provide the very best in medical care for your child. *Preventive medicine, which can keep your child healthy, should always be the main goal and focus.*

To do this, I recommend that all parents find their team of holistic doctors, which should include an osteopathic physician, naturopathic physician and homeopath, to have as their primary medical providers.

Osteopathy, naturopathy and homeopathy can all be used together to provide ongoing health maintenance and to keep your child growing, developing and thriving to his or her full potential. Your child does not need to have any symptoms present to benefit from these treatments.

Osteopathy

As your toddler continues to develop, walk, talk and run, his or her body and brain is going through enormous changes and growth. The osteopath's specialty and expertise is in checking that there is nothing obstructing or interfering with your child's structural development and growth. This includes bones, internal organs, lymphatic system, nervous system and brain. If your child is healthy and all is going well, an osteopathic checkup and treatment every three months can be very helpful. If your child is suffering from any type of symptoms, digestive problems, headaches, recurring ear infections, sleep disturbances or has a developmental disorder or autism, consult with an osteopath and receive ongoing treatments.

Homeopathy

Homeopathic remedies can be given in a constitutional method to provide your child with a remedy that can assist and support his or her development on all levels—physically, emotionally, mentally and spiritually. A skilled homeopath can prescribe one single remedy that your child can take on an ongoing basis to give him or her an extra level of support, protection and wellness. Your child does not need to have any symptoms present for the homeopath to select and prescribe this constitutional remedy. Homeopathic remedies can also be prescribed to treat acute symptoms for coughs, colds, flus and ear infections, as well as for any ongoing conditions such as asthma, eczema, digestive problems, learning disorders, mood and behavioral disorders or autism. Homeopathic treatment is recommended for both health maintenance and to treat any symptoms that may arise at any time.

Naturopathy

The naturopathic doctor works with diet, foods, nutritional supplements, botanical medicine and exercise. We have looked at how important all of these aspects are and how you can provide the best diet and supplements for your child. A naturopathic physician can also treat acute symptoms and more chronic conditions with these modalities. As a parent, you can draw from these fields of medicine to provide your child with medical care that can both improve and maintain health. With these methods of medicine you will be providing your child with treatment that can address and heal the origin of any deeper, ongoing conditions without the side effects and suppression of pharmaceutical drugs.

It's perfectly normal for children to catch a cold, cough or the flu occasionally. But when given the correct natural treatment, they should recover quickly, easily and completely. It is not normal for children to get sick frequently, catch every bug that is going around, or endure long recovery times. It is not normal to suffer from ongoing congestion, mucus or coughs, recurrent ear, sinus or upper respiratory infections. And it is certainly not normal for children to require antibiotics every time they catch something.

Environmental Detoxification and Neutralization

By eating well, eating clean foods, drinking clean water and giving your child the supplements as recommended above, you will automatically be helping to minimize exposure to environmental toxins while also assisting his or her body to detoxify and eliminate any toxins your child may come into contact with.

Dealing with environmental toxicity is a fact of life in today's world. It is also a fact that children are more sensitive and more easily harmed by these pollutants than we are as adults.

By working with a holistic physician you can test, check and monitor your child to see if any of these toxins are accumulating or impacting their health: urine and hair analysis for heavy metals, blood and urine tests for chemicals, and saliva and stool analysis for digestive ecology and function. Screening your child periodically for these substances can be a normal and routine part of health maintenance and prevention.

If these tests indicate that your child is being affected and burdened by any of these substances, it is best to work with your holistic doctor to develop and customize a detoxification program specifically for your child and his or her circumstance.

Exercise

The absolute necessity and importance of exercise cannot be recognized enough. For at least 100,000 years of human evolution, we have depended upon and survived because of our physical prowess and abilities. We cannot change 100,000 years of evolution, dependence and biological history because of 50 years of television, videos, cars and computers. As each generation in the past 50 years has spent more time and grown more dependent on television, video games, computers and cars the world has grown lazier, sicker and more obese.

In his outstanding book *Born to Run*, Christopher McDougall outlines the evolutionary history and science of how human beings evolved because of our ability to breathe and walk, jog or run for longer distances and longer periods of time than any other species on this planet.[8]

Our DNA, our structure, our immune system, our brain, our very health and well-being are totally connected and dependent on exercise to stay in good working order throughout our lives. The blueprint, habits and foundation for this exercise should begin in childhood and continue for the rest of our lives.

The consequences of children not exercising enough are being illustrated by the epidemic of obesity, high blood pressure and diabetes affecting children in so many countries around the world today.[9, 10]

Physical activity, time and presence in the outdoors need to be an integral part of every child's life.

Chapter 10

The Future

What we do today will be reflected in our life tomorrow and on into the future.

As parents, the degree and foundation of health that you create and establish for your children in childhood will form the quality and shape of the vehicle that carries them into the future.

Profession, money, power, relationships, self-growth and spirituality—all of these aspects of life pale in comparison when measured against the importance of health.

Without the vitality and inherent strength that good health provides, every other experience and human endeavor becomes compromised, less enjoyable, less fruitful, less productive, less rewarding—weaker.

Health is the very essence that is at the core of human experience.

The degree of health creates the size and strength of each individual's vessel, determining the size and capacity of our body's, mind's and soul's ability to create, hold and enjoy the experiences that this lifetime can provide.

We are all born into this world with a myriad of possibilities and outcomes waiting to occur and be experienced. Nothing is more powerful in shaping these outcomes and experiences than the influences that you provide to your child in his or her first seven years.

As we grow and move through our lifetime, it is our innermost thoughts, feelings, perceptions and reactions that we all end up spending the most time with. These thoughts, feelings and perceptions exist in our bodies as well as in our minds.

This place of private and silent thoughts, feelings, and perceptions becomes the loudest and most powerful part of how our life unfolds. This quiet but profoundly powerful state of being and health will reflect all the choices you make and provide to your child as he or she grows.

Diet, food, supplementation with vitamins and minerals, detoxification, medical interventions, environmental impacts— these will all shape your child's physical, emotional and mental health. Care, nurturance, love, discipline, guidance, explanations, honesty, wisdom—these are the qualities that will shape your child's spirit and soul.

It is the energy, impressions and effects of this care and experience that are left to reside within each child's body, mind, emotions and soul. The sum total of all these experiences and the degree of health will then contribute profoundly to the life that your child leads and experiences.

We have looked at how many more health challenges exist for children growing up in today's world than for children of previous generations. We have also looked at how to be aware of these challenges and exactly what you can do to provide the best foods, nutrients, natural remedies and holistic medical care for your child. By applying these recommendations, you can ensure that your child's health is protected, nourished and encouraged to develop to his or her full strength and potential.

It does take more time, more education and more effort in this day and age to provide your child with everything needed to be healthy. At the same time, we know that robust health is the most important factor for determining the shape, satisfaction and happiness of this lifetime. There can be no compromise and no shortcuts in doing all that we can do provide the very best start and foundation in life for our children. You, the parents, are the guardians, the ones whose hands and hearts are entrusted with this responsibility and gift.

I thank you for taking the time and care to read this book, and I trust that these thoughts, suggestions and recommendations can play a part in creating and maintaining a lifetime of outstanding health for you and your children.

I found a fruitful world, because my ancestors planted it for me. Likewise I am planting for my children.
*—Talmud, Ta'anit **23a.***

Appendix I

Medical Treatments for Specific Conditions

In this appendix, I have provided treatment suggestions for the most common first-aid situations, acute infections and chronic conditions seen in children. Treatment advice includes dietary, nutritional, herbal and homeopathic recommendations for the following conditions:

Note: *With all homeopathic remedies, the pellets should be placed in your child's mouth without being touched by hand. Encourage your child to allow the pellets to melt and dissolve slowly in the mouth, rather than chewing them. The remedy should always be given at least 15 minutes away from (before or after) any other medication, food or drink.*

Autism, Autistic spectrum, Asperger's syndrome

All of the developmental and autistic spectrum disorders involve different degrees of dysfunction in our most sophisticated and delicate organ: the brain. From the perspective of holistic and biomedical medicine, we know that the brain does not just malfunction by itself. Any malfunction is usually the result of a direct brain injury from trauma and concussion, or the consequences of an ongoing immune/inflammatory reaction that is occurring within the brain and triggered by some form of irritant or external pathogen. In the majority of children suffering from any one of these disorders, a multi-faceted approach is required to address and heal the underlying and associated problems in the body that are directly related to and contributing to the dysfunction of the brain.

Most importantly, healing and curing a child with any of these conditions requires patience and time. In my own clinic, the biggest factor determining the degree of success in curing children with these conditions has been the ability of the parents to consistently apply the treatment and remedies.

This treatment requires a well-organized and comprehensive approach involving each of the following six key components:

- Dietary evaluation and intervention
- Gastrointestinal evaluation and healing
- Nutritional supplementation
- Detoxification of metals and chemicals when necessary
- Osteopathic craniosacral treatment
- Homeopathic constitutional remedy

Dietary intervention: Always start by placing your child on his or her blood type diet and then utilize the ELISA blood allergy test to identify and eliminate any specific food allergens. Further testing for gluten and casein sensitivity can clarify whether you need to apply a casein/gluten-free diet as well.

Tests: Blood type, ELISA allergy blood test, gluten/casein sensitivity stool test

Gastrointestinal evaluation and healing: Dysbiosis (an imbalance in the correct bacterial ecology within the intestines), yeast or fungal overgrowth (often associated with *candida*), the presence of amoeba or parasites, leaky gut syndrome (increased intestinal permeability), biofilm (an accumulation of bio debris and material on the intestinal wall lining).

Any one of these conditions, when present in the intestines, will disrupt the proper absorption and metabolism of nutrients from your child's food. This in turn will prevent your child's brain and body from receiving all the nutrients and fuel they need to grow and function properly.

In addition, when any one of these conditions are present they will also cause ongoing exposure to the toxins and waste products being released from the bacterial, yeast, fungal, parasitic or biofilm accumulation and overgrowth. These toxins create a huge burden on a child's immune system as well as directly affecting, irritating and poisoning the nervous system and brain.

Tests: Comprehensive digestive stool analysis (CDSA), which should include parasitology, bacterial analysis, yeast and fungal analysis, intestinal permeability.

Nutritional Supplementation: To support organ systems and improve metabolic, immunologic and brain function. Vitamins, minerals, amino acids, essential fatty acids, digestive enzymes, probiotics, and specific anti-oxidants can all be given in the appropriate amounts and dosages to help your child's body, brain and immune system repair, recover and return to normal function.

Tests: Blood tests for fatty acid profile, blood tests for vitamins and minerals, urinalysis for amino acid profile.

Detoxification of metals and chemicals when necessary: When testing clearly indicates that your child's system is being obstructed and compromised by specific metal or chemical toxins, the appropriate detoxification strategy should be determined with the help of your health-care professional. Detoxification should be done carefully and only after the other steps outlined above have already been implemented and given time to be effective. *Detoxification without first checking and repairing the barrier systems, which include the intestinal lining and the blood-brain barrier, is not only wrong but very dangerous and will cause far more harm than good. Any toxins released with the detoxification or chelating agents can be immediately reabsorbed and deposited into the body, the organs, and directly into the brain, if these barriers are not repaired correctly first.*

Tests: Urine analysis for heavy metals, hair analysis for heavy metals, organic acid profile for chemicals, blood analysis for chemicals.

Osteopathic craniosacral treatment: Consult with a well-qualified osteopath to evaluate and address the situation. Osteopathic treatments will always be important to assist in condition that involves brain dysfunction. With their sophisticated knowledge of cranial, organ and structural anatomy, the osteopathic techniques for adjusting and aligning the body, nervous system and brain are an essential part of healing and restoring proper brain development and function.

Homeopathic constitutional remedy: Consult with a well-qualified homeopathic physician who can prescribe the single correct constitutional remedy. A single, correct homeopathic remedy has the ability to heal the deepest origins of a child's developmental or autistic disorder. The physical, emotional and mental symptoms are healed from the inside out while simultaneously addressing and healing the deepest aspects of their spiritual afflictions and obstructions.

ADD, ADHD (attention deficit disorder), (attention deficit/ hyperactivity disorder)

Both of these disorders reflect a dysfunction in a child's nervous system and brain. The same multifaceted approach as outlined above is recommended for treating and healing these conditions, too. ADD/ADHD are a relatively milder symptom of brain dysfunction than the autistic spectrum disorders, so they generally require less intervention and less time to correct. However, it is still useful to follow the same approach so that you and your health-care provider can test, determine and apply the correct treatment in exactly the right areas that your child requires.

Air Travel

To help an infant or child relax and sleep during a long flight

- Start with **Bach Rescue Remedy** liquid drops: 2-3 drops by mouth every 30 minutes until you can see that your child has calmed down.

- If this is not enough, give **valerian herbal extract liquid**: 10 drops every hour until you can see signs of relaxation.

- If this is not effective, try **melatonin**: one, 1mg tablet. (Melatonin should only be used on a very occasional basis and should not be used continually.)

For extra immune support and protection against colds, coughs or flu, give the following supplements beginning the day before travel, while traveling and continuing for a few days afterward:

- Elderberry Extract at the suggested label dosage for your child's age.

- Vitamin C: 250-500 mg three times daily.

Allergies, environmental

An environmental allergy (a reaction to pollen, mold, pollutants or chemicals) is a sign that the immune system is not working properly—that the immune system is reacting abnormally to substances that really shouldn't bother it. It behaves like a blindfolded person who cannot discriminate between friend and enemy, so lashes out at everyone and anyone he meets.

Standard allopathic medical diagnosis is made by conducting allergen tests via the blood or skin. Standard medical treatment usually involves suppressing the symptoms by suppressing the immune system with the ongoing use of oral antihistamines, nasal decongestants, steroidal sprays and allergy shots. All of these pharmaceutical medications directly or indirectly suppress and weaken the immune system over time, which is the exact opposite of what actually needs to be done to cure this condition.

The environmental allergy tests are of limited use, as it is impossible to avoid the pollen, dander, dust and grasses that are most associated with environmental allergies. Correcting, strengthening and balancing the malfunctioning immune system is the ultimate cure and should be the objective of any medical treatment.

Homeopathic Treatment:

Consult with a well-qualified homeopathic physician who can prescribe the single correct constitutional homeopathic remedy.

Osteopathic Treatment:

Consult with a well-qualified osteopath to evaluate and address the situation. Osteopathic treatments will always help improve the function of your child's immune system by improving and facilitating the flow of your child's cerebrospinal fluid, lymphatic system and nervous system.

Dietary Treatment:

Underlying food sensitivities or food allergies may contribute to your child's increased sensitivity and susceptibility to environmental allergies. (*See* Chapter 2 on food allergies.) Test for any food allergies and gluten sensitivity and provide your child with the foods that suit his or her blood type.

Herbal Support:

These herbs can be utilized for their anti-inflammatory, antioxidant and immune regulating properties:

- Amla: 500 mg daily
- Elderberry: 500 mg daily
- Larch arabinogalactan: 1 teaspoon daily

Nutritional Supplements:

Supplement with those nutrients that can help regulate the immune system. The primary nutrient that provides anti-inflammatory, antioxidant, and immune regulating properties for allergies is:

- Quercitin: 250-500 mg three times daily

In addition, your child should be taking the following supplements for strengthening and regulating basic immune function:

- Probiotics: 1/3 teaspoon daily
- Colostrum: 1/2-1 teaspoon daily
- Cod liver oil: 1 teaspoon daily
- Vitamin C: 250-500 mg two times daily

Tests:
- Food, gluten and environmental allergy testing
  Stool analysis for any underlying digestive dysfunction

Allergies, food

(*See* Chapter 2: Food Allergies)

The complete approach for identifying, prioritizing and treating food allergies is contained in Chapter 2.

Asthma

Conventional treatment with pharmaceutical drugs such as antihistamines, antibiotics and steroids can manage asthma symptoms but do not provide a cure, and ultimately will lead to the weakening and deterioration of the child's immune system and overall health.[1, 2] If your child is already taking these medications, continue them while implementing the following treatments and wait until your physician determines that you can safely decrease and eliminate the medications.

Treatment for asthma should focus on strengthening your child's immune system, improving lung and respiratory function, while healing and resolving any emotional or spiritual discords. At the same time, it's important to remove any potential obstacles or aggravating factors from the diet or home environment.

Environment:

Clean up the home environment. Typically, the air quality inside a house is four times worse than it is outside. (For a complete discussion of removing environmental allergens, *see* section on environmental allergies in Chapter 2.)

In addition:

- Replace all household cleaners, soaps and detergents with completely biologically safe and chemical-free products.

- Utilize a portable HEPA-filter air cleaner in your house and particularly in your child's bedroom.

- Hardwood floors are always preferable to carpeting but if this is not an option, then vacuum your carpets with a vacuum cleaner equipped with a HEPA filter.

Dietary Treatment:

Eliminate any allergenic foods, test for gluten sensitivity and provide your child with the foods that best suit his or her blood type.[3] (*See* section on diet and allergies in Chapter 1.)

Nutritional Supplements:

- Vitamin C: 250 mg-500 mg two times daily

- Quercitin: 250-500 mg two times daily

- Probiotics: 1/3 teaspoon daily (this should contain the three most important "friendly" bacteria for children: *Bifidobacterium bifidum*, *Bifidobacterium infantis*, and *Lactobacillus acidophilus*).

- Colostrum: 1/2-1 teaspoon daily. (For most children, this is very helpful and can be given every other day. However, if your child's allergy test indicates that he or she is allergic to cow's milk, do not give colostrum, as it may contain small amounts of milk protein.)

- Cod liver oil (1 teaspoon) or flaxseed oil (1 tablespoon). Both of these omega-3 oils can help reduce inflammation throughout the body, including the lungs.

Homeopathic Treatment:

Consult with a well-qualified homeopathic physician who can prescribe the single correct constitutional remedy. A single correct homeopathic remedy has the ability to heal the deepest origins of asthma, including any inherited predispositions, as well as any emotional and mental conflicts that may be causing the asthma.

Osteopathic Treatment:

Consult with a well-qualified osteopath to evaluate and address any structural problems that may be causing or contributing to asthma. Osteopathic manipulation can help improve the function of your child's respiratory, immune and nervous systems.

Tests:

- Food, gluten and environmental allergy testing
- Stool analysis for any underlying digestive dysfunction

Bites (insect, spider)

The severity of the reaction and the medical treatment will depend on the type of spider bite, so try to identify the species, if possible.

Homeopathic Treatment:

Under ideal circumstances, the advice of a homeopathic physician should be sought immediately to determine the proper remedy for your child. However, if this is not possible, start with the following remedies:

- Ledum 30 c: 1 pellet every 3-4 hours (if the area is blue, purple, white, cold)
- Apis Mel 30 c: 1 pellet every 3-4 hours (if the area is red, hot and swollen)

Continue with remedy until all symptoms are resolved.

Nutritional Supplements:

- Quercitin: 250-500 mg three times daily
- Vitamin C: 250-500 mg three times daily

Burns and Sunburn

For any major burns, always seek medical care immediately. For minor burns or sunburn:

Homeopathic Treatment:

- Calendula 30 c: 1 pellet three times daily

- Calendula gel: Apply immediately and liberally to the affected area and reapply at least 4 times daily. Continue until the skin is completely healed.

Colds

The common cold is usually caused by a viral infection that can affect the nasal passages, throat, airways, and lungs. In addition, there may be more systemic symptoms such as body aches, tiredness, dizziness, headache, fever and effects on mood. You can help your child recover more easily and reduce the duration of a cold with the following remedies.[4]

Homeopathic Treatment:

Select one of the following remedies:

- Chamomilla – congested, cough, cranky

- Eupatorium Perf – achy bones, cough, fever

- Ferrum Phos – fever, headache, cough

- Gelsemium – achy muscles, tired, fatigued, fever

- Kali Bichromicum – yellow, green, sticky nasal mucus, irritable

- Mercurius Sol – fever, sweat, bad breath, nasal mucus, sore throat

- Pulsatilla – fever, cough, congested, clingy, wants to be held

Give the remedy in 30 c potency, 1 pellet every 4 hours until all symptoms are clear.

Herbal Support:

- Echinacea: 10-20 drops four times daily

- Elderberry extract: 1 teaspoon four times daily

Nutritional Supplements:

- Vitamin C: 250-500 mg three times daily

- Zinc lozenges: every 4 hours

- Honey: 1/2 teaspoon honey three times daily (ideally Manuka honey)

Drink:

- Hot water with ginger and honey[5]

Coughs

A cough is often the first sign that your child has come in contact with a respiratory bacteria or a virus, and that the body is responding to the challenge. The immune system, bronchial airways and lungs activate immunoglobulins, which stimulate the mucosal tissues to produce immune factors. These, in turn, secrete mucus and fluids to trap the invading bug, which is then expelled, partially through coughing. That's why suppressing a cough is a bad idea. Instead, treatment should be aimed at helping and assisting the body to remove the invading bug so the bronchial passages and lungs can return to normal.

Homeopathic Treatment:

Select one of the following remedies:

- Ferrum Phos – cough with fever and headache

- Rumex Crispus – mucus, wet cough

- Spongia Tosta – dry, barking cough

- Coccus Cacti – spasmodic, irritated, frequent cough

Give the remedy in 30 c potency, 1 pellet every 4 hours until all symptoms are resolved.

Herbal Support:
- Elderberry herbal extract: 1 teaspoon four times daily

Nutritional Supplements:

- Vitamin C: 250-500 mg three times daily

- Honey: 1/2 teaspoon three times daily (ideally buckwheat or Manuka honey)

Drink:

- Hot water, ginger and honey

Cuts, scratches, puncture wounds

For any type of cut, scratch, abrasion or puncture wound that does not require stitches, cleanse thoroughly and irrigate the cut with 3 percent hydrogen peroxide solution to clean any debris and prevent infection. After cleaning, consider the following:

Homeopathic Treatment:

- Calendula 30 c: 1 pellet one to three times daily, depending on the severity

- HyperCal: apply this ointment or gel, which contains hypericum and calendula extracts, at least three times daily until the area is healed. These two herbal extracts can prevent infection and promote the healing of tissue and skin.

If the cut involves a puncture wound, you can also give

- Ledum 30 c: 1 pellet two times daily for 3 days

Digestive Disorders

Colic, constipation, diarrhea, reflux and stomachaches are the most common childhood digestive maladies. If your baby, infant or child has difficulty with any of these symptoms, consult a well-qualified homeopath and a well-qualified osteopath to help you implement the following recommendations.

Homeopathic Treatment:

A homeopathic physician can prescribe the single correct constitutional remedy. Since homeopathic remedies are always dissolved and absorbed in the mouth, they are very practical and easily given to babies and infants of any age.

Osteopathic Treatment:

An osteopath can evaluate and address any structural or nervous problems that may be causing or contributing to the digestive difficulties.

The vagus nerve travels from the brain all the way down the chest and into the abdominal organs. This nerve is the connection between the brain, the nervous system and the digestive system. Osteopaths can directly and effectively treat this whole system with their techniques.

Dietary Treatment:

If you are unable to breastfeed and are using formula, consider using the following types:

- **Select the best formula that suits your baby's blood type**. (*See* Chapter 1.)

- **Partially hydrolyzed milk protein formula**. This is milk protein that has been broken down into smaller particles, making it easier to digest, assimilate and metabolize. It's ideal for babies with colic, gassiness, constipation or diarrhea. In the United States the primary formula in this category is Good Start.

- **Hypoallergenic formulas.** These formulas have been extensively hydrolyzed and are designed for babies who are highly allergic or have severe digestive difficulties. In the United States, these include Nutramigen, Pregestamiland Alimentum. Generally, these specialty formulas should be suggested and prescribed by a pediatrician.

Once you start to introduce solid foods, use your child's blood type to guide you in choosing the foods that will suit him or her best. (See Chapter 1.)

Nutritional Supplements:

- **Probiotics:** 1/3 teaspoon daily (this should contain the three most important "good" bacteria for children: *Bifidobacterium bifidum, Bifidobacterium infantis, Lactobacillus acidophilus*).[6, 7]

- **Colostrum:** 1/2 -1 teaspoon daily (for most children, this is very useful and can be given every other day. However, if your child's allergy test indicates that he or she is allergic to cow's milk, do not give colostrum as it may contain small amounts of milk protein).

- **Cod liver oil:** 1 teaspoon, **or flaxseed oil:** 1 tablespoon. (Both of these omega-3 oils can help reduce inflammation within the digestive tract and also help to re-establish the correct ecology flora and fauna within the gut.)

Tests:

- Food allergy and gluten sensitivity test

- Stool analysis for complete digestive evaluation, including

  - dysbiosis (an imbalance or deficiency in the "friendly," normal, good bacteria that are present in a healthy digestive system)

  - bacterial overgrowth and infections

  - yeast overgrowth (most common, *candida*)

  - fungal infections

  - parasitic infestations

An excellent lab for testing and evaluating intestinal function and stool analysis is Diagnos-Techs Inc., located in Washington state, and found at www.diagnostechs.com

Fever

A fever is a healthy and appropriate response to an invading "bug." The increase in body temperature triggers a cascade of immune and physiological responses that create a powerful immune system surge. Suppress the fever and you will dampen the immune system's ability to respond appropriately and effectively. In the short term, this will slow your child's recovery from the infection. In the long term, it will interfere with the full growth and maturation of your child's immune system.

The correct treatment for fever is to give the remedies and nutrients that will support and assist the immune response. This will ensure that the invading organism is located, killed and completely cleared from the body, and that antibodies are created by the immune system to ward off any future encounters with the same or a similar bug.

Homeopathic Treatment:

The following remedies work by supporting the immune response and helping to overcome (but not suppress) the fever. Select one:

- Aconitum – sudden, quick-onset chills/fever

- Belladonna – intense fever, headache, red face, cold hands, delirious

- Chamomilla – fever, cranky, irritable, inconsolable

- Ferrum Phos – fever, headache

- Pulsatilla – fever, clingy, crying, wants to be held all the time

Give the remedy in 30 c potency, 1 pellet every 4 hours until all symptoms are resolved.

Herbal Support:
- Echinacea: 10-20 drops four times daily

Nutritional Supplements:

- Vitamin C: 250-500 mg three times daily

- Zinc lozenges every 4 hours

Drink:

- Hot water with lemon, ginger and honey

Flu (influenza)

The influenza viruses are usually stronger than the viruses that trigger the common cold. Symptoms of flu may include fever/chills, fatigue, nasal congestion, coughing, sneezing, eye sensitivity, headache, body aches, nausea and vomiting. It is not unusual for your child's appetite to decrease while fighting the infection. However, it's important to make sure that he or she takes in enough fluids to stay well-hydrated.

The severity of flu symptoms and the recovery time can be improved with the following:

Homeopathic Treatment:

Select one of the following remedies:

- Ferrum Phos – fever, headache, cough

- Gelsemium – chills/fever, muscle ache, tired, fatigued, dizzy

- Eupatorium Perf – fever, bones ache, cough

- Arsenicum album – watery mucus, stomach upset, restless

- Belladonna – fever, red face, cold hands, delirious

- Aconitum – sudden onset, chills/fever, pale, scared

- Chamomilla – chills/fever, congested, cranky, irritable

Give the remedy in 30 c potency, 1 pellet every 4 hours until all symptoms are resolved.

Herbal Support:

- Elderberry Extract at the suggested label dosage for your child's age; or

- Echinacea : 10-20 drops four times daily

Nutritional Supplements:

- Vitamin C: 250-500 mg three times daily

- Zinc lozenges every 4 hours

Drink:

- Hot water with lemon, ginger and honey (every 4 hours)

Flu, stomach

Stomach flu may be due to either bacterial or viral infection, and with acute onset it can cause fever, nausea, abdominal pain, diarrhea and vomiting. Because of fluid loss due to vomiting and/ or diarrhea, it is important to keep your child well-hydrated, preferably via a healthy electrolyte-containing drink such as Nature's One, PediaVance formula, which is made with all-organic ingredients.

Homeopathic Treatment:

Select one of the following remedies:

- Gelsemium – nausea, diarrhea, body/muscle aches, tired, fatigued

- Arsenicum album – nausea, vomiting, diarrhea, restless

- Veratrum album – vomiting, diarrhea, chills

Give the remedy in 30 c potency, 1 pellet every 4 hours, until all symptoms are resolved.

Herbal Support:

It is better not to use any herbal remedies in this situation as the herbs will not be absorbed well and can further irritate the digestive tract.

Nutritional Supplements:

- **Probiotics**: 1/3 teaspoon daily (this should contain the three most important "friendly" bacteria for children: *Bifidobacterium bifidum*, *Bifidobacterium infantis*, and *Lactobacillus acidophilus*).[6, 7]

- **Colostrum:** 1/2-1 teaspoon daily (for most children, this will be very useful. However, if your child's allergy test indicates that he or she is allergic to cow's milk, do not give colostrum as it may contain small amounts of milk protein).

Drink:

- Ginger tea every 4 hours

- Electrolyte formula: as needed to replace fluids lost from vomiting or diarrhea. (Preferably, use a healthy electrolyte-containing drink such as Nature's One, PediaVance formula, which is made with all-organic ingredients.)

Food Poisoning

This results from eating food that has spoiled or been contaminated with some type of bug, and usually occurs within 48 hours of eating the contaminated food. Symptoms can include stomach and abdominal pain, nausea, chills, fever, vomiting and/or diarrhea.

Homeopathic Treatment:

- Arsenicum album 30 c: give 1 pellet every 2-4 hours depending on the severity of the symptoms. Continue until all symptoms are clear.

Hypoglycemia, reactive

Reactive hypoglycemia is a condition in which abnormal fluctuations in insulin and cortisol levels cause blood sugar to drop dramatically 2-4 hours after meals. These abnormal insulin and cortisol levels usually result from the consumption of too much sugar and other refined carbohydrates, and/or engaging in irregular eating habits (e.g., missing meals).

Symptoms can include fatigue, anxiety, headaches, difficulty concentrating, sweaty palms, shakiness, excessive hunger, drowsiness, abdominal pain, moodiness and depression. Clinically, the symptoms of hypoglycemia include post-meal blood levels (2-4 hours after a meal) of 85 mg/dl or less of glucose.

Dietary Treatment:

Hypoglycemia can be greatly improved and corrected by making healthy changes in food choices and dietary habits. Eliminate refined sugars and ensure that each meal contains at least 30 percent protein intake (meats, poultry, fish, eggs, cheese) along with carbohydrates, which have a low glycemic rating and are high in fiber (whole grains, fruits, vegetables, legumes, nuts). Include healthy fats and oils (olive oil, sunflower oil, flaxseed oil, butter).[9]

Provide your child with the foods that best suit his or her blood type. (*See section on diet and blood type in Chapter 1.*)

Nutritional Supplements:

- Key nutrients to consider are those that assist insulin regulate blood sugar levels. They include:

- Chromium: 25-100 mcg daily[10]

- Magnesium: 150-300 mg daily[11]

- Niacinamide (vitamin B3): 25-35 mg daily[12]

- Cod liver oil: 1 teaspoon daily[13]

- Probiotics: 1/3 teaspoon daily

- Multivitamin/mineral: follow recommended serving size for your child's age[14]

Tests:

- Food allergy and gluten-sensitivity testing
- Stool analysis for digestive function

Homeopathic Treatment:

Consult with a well-qualified homeopathic physician who can prescribe the single correct constitutional remedy and assist you in correcting your child's eating patterns.

Infection, ear

Otitis media is the formal name for inflammation and infection within the middle ear. Infants and children are more susceptible to ear infections due to the size and structure of the young ear cavity and the surrounding lymphatic drainage system. The infection may be associated with fever, congestion, fussiness, crankiness and pain in or around the ear.

Homeopathic Treatment:

Consult with a well-qualified homeopathic physician who can prescribe a remedy to treat the acute infection and symptoms, as well as prescribe the single correct constitutional remedy, which can then be taken on an ongoing basis to help reduce the susceptibility to recurring ear infections.

The remedy to treat the acute symptoms and infection may be one of the following; select one:

- Chamomilla – cranky, crying, inconsolable mood
- Pulsatilla – crying, clingy, wants to be held, inconsolable
- Belladonna – fever, red face, painful, restless
- Mercurius sol – sweaty, ear discharge, odor, lethargic

Give the appropriate remedy in 30 c potency, 1 pellet every 4 hours until all symptoms are clear.

Herbal Support:

- Echinacea at the suggested label dosage for your child's age

Nutritional Supplements:

- Vitamin C: 250-500 mg three times daily
- Zinc lozenges every 4 hours

Drink:

- Hot water with lemon and honey, every 4 hours

Ear Drops:

- Mullein oil ear drops, every 4 hours[15]

Osteopathic Treatment:

See a well-qualified osteopathic physician who can carefully adjust the structures around your child's ear, unblocking any congestion or lymphatic obstruction that can help treat the acute infection, as well as correct any condition that may be contributing to the recurring infection(s).

Dietary Treatment:

Remove all cow products from your child's diet, including cow milk, cow cheese, yogurt and ice cream. Replace with goat milk, goat cheese, goat yogurt and rice ice cream.

Infection, sinus

The major symptoms of a sinus infection are nasal congestion and obstruction due to mucus (which may be clear, yellow or green), facial pain, frontal headache, and sometimes a post-nasal drip that can cause throat irritation and a cough. Acute sinus infections are usually associated with a bacterial infection.

Homeopathic Treatment:

Select one of the following remedies:

- Kali bichromicum – thick yellow, green mucus, irritable mood

- Mercurius sol – yellowish mucus, throat pain, bad breath

- Dulcamara – very congested, blocked nose

Give the appropriate remedy in 30 c potency, 1 pellet every 4 hours until all symptoms are resolved.

Herbal Support:

- Echinacea/Goldenseal: 10-20 drops four times daily
- Elderberry herbal extract: 1 teaspoon four times daily

Nutritional Supplements:

- Vitamin C: 250-500 mg three times daily
- Zinc lozenges every 4 hours

Drink:

- Hot water with lemon, ginger and honey

Infection, throat (sore throat)

A sore throat may be associated with a bacterial or viral infection. It may stand alone or be associated with other conditions such as a cold, sinus infection, the flu and so on.

Homeopathic Treatment:

Select one of the following:

- Phytolacca – throat feels hot, painful, pain radiates to ear when swallowing
- Hepar sulf – very sharp, sticking pain, as if a splinter is stuck in throat
- Mercurius sol – sweaty, bad breath

- Lachesis – swelling, left-sided pain, pain worse when swallowing liquid

- Gelsemium – sore throat with achiness, tiredness and fatigue

Give the appropriate remedy in 30 c potency, 1 pellet every 4 hours until all symptoms are resolved.

Herbal Support:
- Echinacea/Goldenseal: 10-20 drops four times daily[16]

Nutritional Supplements:
- Vitamin C: 250-500 mg three times daily
- Zinc lozenges every 4 hours

Drink:
- Hot water with lemon, ginger and honey (every 4 hours)

Infection, upper respiratory

The symptoms of an upper respiratory infection are similar to those associated with a cold, cough, flu or sinus infection. While they may look the same and affect the same areas, for some reason medical doctors like to give different names to what amounts to essentially the same conditions. Thus, sinusitis, laryngitis, pharyngitis and bronchitis can all be part of an upper respiratory infection.

Treatment for these symptoms will be the same as suggested for colds, coughs, flu or sinus conditions, focusing on the area where the predominant symptoms reside.

Homeopathy Treatment:

Select one of the following remedies:

- Ferrum phos – cough, fever, headache

- Rumex crispus – wet, mucus, cough

- Spongia tosta – dry barking cough

- Coccus cacti – spasmodic, irritated, frequent cough

- Eupatorium perf – cough, fever, achy bones

- Pulsatilla – cough, congested, clingy, wants to be held

Give in 30 c potency, 1 pellet every 4 hours until all symptoms are resolved.

Herbal Support:

- Elderberry herbal extract: 1 teaspoon four times daily

Nutritional Supplements:

- Vitamin C: 250-500 mg three times daily

- Honey: 1/2 teaspoon three times daily (ideally, Manuka honey)

Drink:

- Hot water with lemon, ginger and honey, every 4 hours

Injuries, body (bumps, bruises, sprains and strains)

For any type of bruising injury where there may be swelling, discomfort, discoloration and some post-traumatic fright:

Homeopathic Treatment:

- Arnica 30 c: 1 pellet three times daily until bruising and discomfort is gone

Injuries, head and face (bumps, bruises, concussion)

Homeopathic Treatment:

- Arnica 30 c: 1 pellet three times daily until all bruising or swelling is all clear

If the bump or injury is severe enough to cause a concussion, also give

- Natrum sulphuricum 30 c and Hypericum 30 c: 1 pellet of each, three times daily, in addition to the Arnica

Give all of these remedies daily until all signs of the bruise, concussion or shock are completely gone.

Note: *When giving two or more remedies like this, first give the Arnica pellet, letting it fully dissolve in your child's mouth, then give the Natrum sulphuricum pellet, and then follow with the Hypericum.*

Skin irritation, inflammation or rash (eczema, dermatitis)

The body has its own priority system for protecting us, developing symptoms and preserving life. At the top of the list as most important organ and tissue in the body is the brain. Next in order of importance are the internal organs like the liver, kidneys and lungs, then the nerves, blood vessels, muscles, mucus membranes, and finally, the skin. The skin is our outermost tissue/organ and therefore, the least important in terms of the body's priority system. You can scratch it, cut it, peel it off from sunburn and none of this is at all life-threatening. However, if one tiny cut forms, or one blood vessel breaks in our brain, we can suddenly lose complete function of one side of our body.

When thrown off balance, the body will always try to protect itself by producing symptoms in the least important tissue/organ first. Therefore, very often a skin rash, dermatitis or eczema may be the first sign that something is not quite right with your child as a whole.

The worst treatment that can be applied to any skin condition is suppression with a topical steroid ointment or similar, because it suppresses the symptom, blocks the body's cry for help and does not in any way address the underlying reason for the inflammation or condition. Unfortunately, standard medical treatment for most skin disorders consists of the topical application of some form of cortisone steroid cream or similar. However, this approach does nothing to address the origins of the condition, and only pushes the inflammation deeper inside your child's body. If this misguided treatment goes on long enough and the inflammation continues to be pushed into the body, your child will eventually develop other, deeper symptoms which can manifest as allergies, asthma, recurrent infections or emotional and nervous disorders, depending on where the inflammation is pushed and settles.

Treating any type of skin disorder requires maintaining a delicate balance between easing the symptoms of skin irritation and itchiness without suppressing the inflammation or pushing it deeper into the body. The following treatments can help you to actually heal the condition without suppressing.

Homeopathic Treatment:

Consult with a well-qualified homeopathic physician who can prescribe the single correct constitutional remedy that will address the origin and genesis of the condition and treat it from the inside out. Over time, the symptoms will decrease and clear completely, without any suppression. This usually takes time and is not an overnight event.

Dietary Treatment:

Test for gluten sensitivity. Test and eliminate any allergenic foods and provide your child with the foods that best suit his or her blood type. (*See section on diet and allergies in Chapter 2.*) Food allergies are not usually the sole cause of dermatitis or eczema; however, they can trigger and aggravate the condition and symptoms.

Nutritional Supplements:

- **Probiotics:** 1/3 teaspoon daily (this should contain the three most important "friendly" bacteria for children: *Bifidobacterium bifidum*, *Bifidobacterium infantis*, *Lactobacillus acidophilus*)

- **Colostrum:** 1/2-1 teaspoon daily (for most children, this is very useful when given every other day. However, if your child's allergy test indicates that he or she is allergic to cow's milk, do not give colostrum as it may contain small amounts of milk protein).

- **Cod liver oil:** 1 teaspoon daily, or **flaxseed oil:** 1 tablespoon daily (both of these omega-3 oils can help reduce inflammation throughout the body, including the skin)

Topical Treatment:

It is best not to use any type of ointment long term that will suppress the inflammation. To keep the skin moist and nourished, consider using one of the following or alternating between them:

- Almond oil
- Jojoba oil
- Evening primrose oil

Thicker ointments whose purpose is to primarily coat the skin and maintain moisture can be used as needed. These are usually best applied over and after the oils mentioned above have been absorbed.

Tests:

- Food allergy and gluten sensitivity testing
- Stool analysis for complete digestive evaluation

Many times, there is an associated digestive dysfunction that contributes to our directly causing the skin problems.

Stings, insect

For bee, wasp, or hornet stings:

Homeopathic Treatment:

- Ledum 30 c – 1 pellet three to four times daily
- Apis mel 30 c – 1 pellet three to four times daily
- Carbolic acid 30 c – 1 pellet three to four times daily

Continue to give until all swelling and discomfort is gone

Sunstroke

Sunstroke, sometimes called heatstroke, occurs when the body's heat control system fails and it cannot lose the excessive heat. High temperatures can cause the body's major organs to fail, and this is a potentially life-threatening condition for which medical help should be sought immediately.

In the early stages, the skin may become both hot and dry.

Sweating usually stops, and breathing may become rapid. The body's temperature, along with the pulse, will begin to rise rapidly. Other symptoms include muscle cramps and headaches, a red face, irritability and possible mental and verbal confusion.

Homeopathic Treatment:

- Belladonna 30 c – 1 pellet every hour until improvement is noted, and then every 3-4 hours until temperature, energy and mood have all returned to normal.

Teething

Depending on the nature of each infant and the amount of teeth that may be coming through at any one time, teething can cause irritation, discomfort and pain to your baby, which can translate into a crying, irritable and inconsolable baby.

Homeopathic Treatment:

- Chamomilla 30 c – 1 pellet as needed until some relief is visible and then give 1 pellet three to four times daily while the teething is going on.

Appendix II

Rating the Vaccines

The only wholly safe vaccine is the vaccine that is never used.
—Dr. J. Shannon, National Institutes of Health,
June 23, 1955

Following is an explanation of the most common vaccines currently in use, with an assessment of the degree of risk they each pose to your child.

Again, I do not think that there is such a thing as a completely safe vaccine. There are no scientific studies that any doctor can show you to prove that any vaccine is completely safe. Despite the 50 to 60 years of ongoing vaccine programs, there have been no double-blind, placebo-controlled studies ever conducted on the issue of vaccine ingredients, individual vaccines or multiple vaccine safety. Every other allopathic medical medication, drug or treatment is supposed to go through the scrutiny and evaluation of the double-blind, placebo-controlled trials…why not vaccinations, too?

There is information, documentation and statistics on adverse vaccine reactions available at the National Vaccine Information Center NVIC www.nvic.org (an informed, parent-run organization that does a masterful job of providing impeccable information on vaccine safety issues). There is also information available at the Vaccine Adverse Event Reporting System www.vaers.hhs.gov (the U.S. government system for tracking adverse vaccine reactions), where it is conservatively estimated that only 10 percent of adverse reactions are actually reported to this database by M.D. pediatricians[1] and from the U.S. government National Vaccine Injury Compensation Program (VICP) at www.hrsa.gov/Vaccinecompensation/

Personally, I continue to look at the big picture and ask this straightforward question: *After 50 years of mass vaccination programs and campaigns, are the children of today healthier than they were 50 years ago?*

The answer is a resounding NO.

Fifty years ago, 1 in every 50 American children suffered from some form of chronic medical disease. Today, 1 out of every 5 American children now suffer with some type of chronic medical disorder.[2]

Within this appendix, I give you an overview of the risk factors associated with each of the vaccines relative to each other. Each of these vaccines has been given a risk rating on a scale of one to four, based on its history of use and potential for adverse reactions.

DTaP: (DIPTHERIA, TETANUS, ACELLULAR PERTUSSIS)

DTaP is a combination (multivalent) vaccine against diphtheria, tetanus and pertussis. DTaP is often given at 2 months, 4 months and 6 months of age along with two other vaccines, Hib (Haemophilus influenzae) and IPV (inactivated polio), at the same office visit. To me, this injection and administration of three, four and five vaccines at one time into a baby barely into this world is frightening, disturbing and completely reckless. It displays a callous disregard for the delicate balance of health and development taking place within a newborn child. Now, let's take a look at the individual components of the DTaP vaccine.

Diptheria is a bacterial infection that affects the upper respiratory tract, causing fever, fatigue, sore throat, and sometimes swelling of the lymph nodes in the neck. Often referred to as the disease of poverty and poor sanitation, diptheria can be fatal, depending on the quality of medical care available. In the United States, however, there have been no fatalities from diphtheria in children under the age of 5 during the past eight years. The last two diphtheria cases in the U.S. were reported in 1998 and 2003, and both occurred in elderly patients.[3]

It is estimated that 85 percent of American children receive the diphtheria vaccine, which was first introduced in 1949. This leaves approximately 15 percent who do not receive this vaccine and who do not catch diphtheria.[4]

Tetanus is a bacterial infection that causes muscular spasms, stiffness and its characteristic symptom "lockjaw," all of which are due to the toxin excreted by the tetanus bacteria. Tetanus is not usually a fatal infection.

The tetanus vaccine is routinely given when a child or adult suffers a cut or puncture wound, although it is extremely rare for these wounds to lead to a tetanus infection. In fact, since the year 2000, only one case of tetanus has been reported in U.S. children under the age of 5, and there have been no fatalities.[5]

The latest figures show that 83 percent of American children receive the tetanus vaccine. Thus, there are approximately 17 percent who do not receive the vaccine and have not caught tetanus.

Pertussis, which is commonly known as whooping cough, is an infection caused by the *Bordatella pertussis* bacteria. Initial symptoms include a cough, nasal congestion, sneezing and sometimes, fever. The cough then becomes more pronounced, with ongoing fits of "whooping cough." The duration of the recovery period may be one to two months.

The most recent data shows there were 5,796 cases of pertussis reported in the United States in 2004 in children under the age of 5 years. In 2003, there were 3,355 cases. The year 2002 showed 3,700 cases. Previous years show an average of around 2,800 occurrences, with 2,878 in the year 2000.

Of the 2,878 cases in 2000, 17 deaths were reported.[6] This author could not find any mortality numbers for subsequent years.

This is not usually a fatal infection, especially when good medical care is available. In New Zealand, where some 20 percent of the population does not receive the vaccine, there were no deaths from pertussis in the years 1988 to 1995, and one death per year was reported from 1999 to 2004.[7]

For many years, a form of the vaccine called DTP, which contained the whole cells of the pertussis bacteria, combined the diphtheria, tetanus and pertussis vaccines into a single shot. In 1991, a book titled *A Shot in the Dark*, by authors Harris Coulter and Barbara Fisher-Loe, exposed the injuries, adverse reactions, lifelong disabilities and deaths due to vaccinations.[8] Of particular concern were the severe adverse reactions associated with the pertussis component of the DTP vaccine. Low-grade, chronic encephalitis (inflammation of the brain) leading to seizures, convulsions, learning disabilities and SIDS (sudden infant death syndrome) have all been caused by this component of the DPT vaccine.[9]

Despite pharmaceutical and medical denials that there were any problems with the DPT vaccine, eventually the pertussis P (whole cell) component was removed and replaced with the acellular pertussis (aP) component.[9] This means that the vaccine is now made from a partial piece of the cells of the bacteria, which has decreased the number of severe and adverse reactions associated with this portion of the vaccine.

However, there is still the problem of three vaccines being combined into one. Diptheria and pertussis vaccines are not available separately and are always injected together. Combination (multivalent) vaccines mean increased genetic material, adjuvants, preservatives and chemical stabilizers, and a greater chance of contaminants. This translates to increased confusion in an infant's immune system and a greater toxic load for the brain and body to neutralize, detoxify and eliminate. Thus, this vaccine belongs to the highest-risk category.

Vaccine Rating - DTaP

****Highest-risk category – DTaP is only available as a combined (multivalent) vaccine, which automatically puts it in the highest-risk category. Never give your child a multivalent vaccine, which exponentially increases the risk of brain and immune system damage.

(The tetanus component of this vaccine is available separately.)

FLU (INFLUENZA)

Influenza is a normal childhood infection with symptoms that include fever, chills, headache, body aches, fatigue, cough and sometimes digestive upsets such as nausea, vomiting and diarrhea. Recovery typically occurs within 3-10 days. It is extremely rare for any complications or fatalities to occur in those who do not already suffer from a chronic underlying medical condition. To illustrate this point, consider the following:

- Of the 73 million children who lived in the United States in 2004, 153 died from influenza, 40 percent of whom were reported to have chronic underlying medical conditions.[10] An estimated 48 percent of American children received the influenza vaccine that year, which means that 36.5 million children did not receive the vaccine and 99.9999 percent of them were okay.

- Of the 1 million children who lived in New Zealand in 2007, none died from influenza. An estimated 30 percent received the flu vaccine, which means that 70 percent or 665,000 children who did not receive the vaccine were still okay.[11]

- Of the 4 million children who lived in Australia in 2007, there were only 6 deaths from influenza reported. The influenza vaccine is not a part of the routine vaccine schedule in Australia; it is usually given only to children with some chronic underlying medical condition. Thus, more than 3 million Australian children do not receive the influenza vaccine and 99.99 percent did not suffer any serious consequence from the flu.[12]

In spite of this, a new vaccine is developed each year containing the flu viruses that researchers believe will be circulating that season. In the United States, the vaccine is routinely administered to infants and children at the beginning of the winter season. Shockingly, some forms of this vaccine still contain thimerosal, a mercury preservative that the FDA requested be removed from all vaccines in 2000.[13] All mercury compounds carry an extremely toxic potential and there is no way of pre-determining which children will be severely affected by thimerosal. Side effects from thimerosal include brain damage and autism.

Vaccine Rating - Influenza Vaccine

****Highest risk category – Some brands of influenza vaccine still contain thimerosal preservative. There is also a contamination risk. Don't allow your child to receive this vaccine. Influenza has been successfully and easily treated for centuries by homeopathic and naturopathic physicians.[14]

HEPATITIS A

Hepatitis A is a viral infection that causes inflammation of the liver. The virus is spread by eating food contaminated with human fecal matter from an infected person, and can be completely prevented by proper hand washing after going to the bathroom or handling diapers. Transference of the virus from one child to another is extremely uncommon. Symptoms include fatigue, fever, jaundice and abdominal pain. The infection is almost always self-curing with no long-term adverse consequences. According to Hepatitis Foundation International, "Hepatitis A will clear up on its own in a few weeks or months with no serious after effects." In young children, 70 percent of cases are completely asymptomatic, meaning the immune system handles the infection without the development of any symptoms.[15]

In 2003 and 2004, before the use of the hepatitis A vaccine in infants and children became routine, 256 cases of the disease were seen in U.S. children on average.[16] This means that of the 70 million children in the U.S., most were not vaccinated against hepatitis A, and there were only 256 cases of the disease, none of which were fatal.

In 2005, the vaccine was included into the routine vaccine schedule in the United States and it is now routinely injected at age 1 with a follow-up dose before age 2. The hepatitis A vaccine is not routinely administered to children in other countries, including New Zealand and Australia.[17, 18]

Vaccine Rating - Hepatitis A

*** High risk category – This rating is elevated to highest risk if hepatitis A vaccine is administered during the same office visit with other vaccines (as is often done at the age 1 visit).

HEPATITIS B

Like hepatitis A, **hepatitis B** is a viral infection that causes inflammation of the liver. However, it is transmitted by direct contact with an infected person's blood, usually via intravenous drug use or extreme sexual promiscuity. Hepatitis B is not life threatening, and 95 percent of all cases recover completely within 3-4 weeks.[19] The rate of recovery can be assisted and improved with homeopathic and nutritional treatment.

Introduced in 1981, the hepatitis B vaccine is now the first one routinely given to newborn babies in the hospital, just 12 hours after birth. Conventional vaccine schedules call for three hepatitis B shots: one at birth, one at 2 months and one at 6 months of age.

The hepatitis B vaccine has been directly linked to juvenile diabetes and severe autoimmune and neurological disorders such as rheumatoid arthritis, lupus and multiple sclerosis [20], with studies conducted and published in Canada and France confirming these effects.[21] As a result, in July of 1998, attorneys representing 15,000 French citizens filed a lawsuit against the French government, accusing government officials of understating the vaccine's risks and exaggerating its benefits for the average person. In October of 1998, the French government responded by stopping all school-based hepatitis B vaccination programs.[21]

In the United States, 872 serious adverse events in children under 14 years of age who had been injected with the hepatitis B vaccine were reported to the Vaccine Adverse Event Reporting System (VAERS) in 1996. The children were either taken to the emergency room, developed life-threatening health problems, were hospitalized, or were left disabled following vaccination. Two hundred and fourteen of the children had received the hepatitis B vaccine alone, while the rest had received the hepatitis B vaccine in combination with other vaccines. Forty-eight children were reported to have died after they were injected with hepatitis B vaccine that year, and 13 of these children had received the hepatitis B vaccine by itself before their deaths.[22]

Between the years 1990 and 1998, VAERS logged a total of 24,775 hepatitis-B-vaccine-related adverse events, including 9,673 serious adverse events and 439 deaths. These are frightening numbers, especially when it is conservatively estimated that only 10 percent of all vaccine-related adverse events and reactions are actually reported by pediatricians to the VAERS system.[22]

In New Zealand, the hepatitis B vaccine was introduced in 1988, with vaccination beginning at 6 weeks of age. Research has revealed that within 3 years of the introduction of this vaccine, New Zealand suffered a 60 percent increase in the number of children diagnosed with insulin-dependent type 1 diabetes.[23] Dr. Classens, a former researcher at the U.S. National Institutes of Health who spearheaded this research, concluded that increasing the number of vaccines that children receive and vaccinating at such a young age induces immune-mediated diabetes. His research showed that there can be a one-to-four-year time period between the time the vaccine is given and the onset of type 1 diabetes in children.

Vaccine Rating - Hepatitis B

**** Highest risk category – This vaccine is directly linked to juvenile diabetes and severe autoimmune and neurological disorders such as rheumatoid arthritis, lupus and multiple sclerosis. Also, incredibly, some forms of this vaccine (e.g., Recombivax) still include the mercury preservative thimerosal (which has shown to lead to brain damage and autism).

Hib (HAEMOPHILUS INFLUENZAE TYPE B)

Haemophilus is a type of bacteria that can cause meningitis (inflammation of the protective membranes covering the spine and brain stem) in infants and children. Meningitis is usually associated with a fever, headache and stiffness in the neck. Meningitis can lead to serious long-term consequences such as deafness, epilepsy and impaired brain development, especially if not treated quickly.

The Haemophilus influenza type B (Hib) vaccine is made from part of the bacteria's cell wall. A relative newcomer (it was licensed and added to the vaccine schedule in 1985), Hib is routinely injected at 2 months, 4 months and 12 months. Although it is available as an individual vaccine, it is usually given at the same time as the DTaP, (diphtheria, tetanus, pertussis), IPV (polio) and PCV (pneumococcal) vaccines.

Hib infection causing meningitis is uncommon in children over the age of 5 years and the fatality rate from this infection is around 5 percent. The latest U.S. statistics show that there were 331 cases of meningitis resulting in 15 fatalities in the year 2004.[24] In New Zealand, where there is an estimated 80 percent vaccination compliance rate, there were two cases of meningitis that year: one had received the Hib vaccination; the other had not. Around 180,000 New Zealand children (20 percent) are not vaccinated against Hib.[25] With two cases of Hib infection in the whole country and one of them developing in a child who *was* vaccinated, this means that just 1 unvaccinated child out of 180,000 actually developed the infection.

In the United States, approximately 15 million children are not vaccinated against Hib.[26] With 331 cases of Hib meningitis in 2004, this means one child in 45,000 caught Hib meningitis and 1 in 1,000,000 died from it. Statistics like these are often impersonal, distant and cold; however, they are useful for putting the risks versus the benefits of a given vaccine in perspective.

Of course, whether or not a child will develop a viral or bacterial infection will ultimately be determined by the strength of his or her immune system, current nutritional status, and various environmental and emotional stressors. Approximately 50 percent of all children have the *Haemophilus* bacteria present in their noses and throats without any symptoms being present.[27] These children's immune systems are able to handle the bacteria without any problem. Therefore, when deciding what is best for your child, keep in mind that a strong, healthy immune system is the ultimate defense against any type of infection.

Vaccine rating – Hib

**Medium risk category – When given individually, this vaccine carries a medium risk. However, it increases to highest risk if injected at the same time as DTaP, IPV and PCV vaccines due to the accumulative toxic and immune burden.

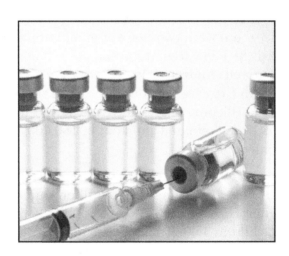

MMR (MEASLES, MUMPS AND RUBELLA)

Measles, mumps and rubella (German measles) are viral infections that cause various symptoms: fever, cold symptoms and a rash in measles; swelling in the salivary glands of the cheeks, sore throat and fever in mumps; and fever and a rash in rubella. Complications or fatalities from any of these diseases are extremely rare (less than 0.1 percent).

Vaccines were introduced against measles in 1963, mumps in 1967, rubella in 1969 and the combined MMR was introduced in 1971. The live virus MMR vaccine, which is still routinely used, was introduced in 1973. Up until these vaccines were developed, measles, mumps, and rubella were considered normal childhood illnesses. No big deal. Suddenly, the pharmaceutical industry turned these normal childhood occurrences into "life-threatening" illnesses that all children must be vaccinated against. I remember when my sister and I caught measles. We got to stay home from school, were looked after by our mother, played cards, sat in front of the fire, ate lots of soup and received lots of loving care. It was ultimately a good experience that I remember to this day.

What turned these normal childhood illnesses into deadly diseases? In reality, nothing. They are the same viruses that they have always been. Indeed, you can safely argue that catching these normal childhood illnesses is an important—even essential part of developing a strong immune system that will look after us well for the rest of our lives.

While the risks of long-term consequences and fatalities from catching any of these infections are extremely low, the same cannot be said about the risks of this multivalent vaccine. The MMR vaccine has been strongly implicated in the development of autistic symptoms in many children, although this has been continuously denied by vaccine manufacturers and many in the allopathic medical community.[28] However, there are too many parents and doctors who have seen and experienced the onset of autism in children after receiving this vaccine. I have listened to mothers tell me firsthand what happened to their previously normal children after they received their first MMR vaccine.

Live viral vaccines always carry the highest degree of risk of adverse effects. Not only is the child exposed to the virus, but it is injected directly into his or her body, bypassing all the normal immune barriers that the immune system utilizes for identifying and responding to viruses before they penetrate internally. The combination live viral vaccines are the worst. In the natural world, it would be extremely unusual for a child to be exposed to the measles, mumps, and rubella viruses all at once, in the same moment, on the same day. And yet, the MMR vaccine does just that to a 12-month-old infant. Along with the live viruses, the infant faces the additional toxic burden of the chemical preservatives, adjuvants and stabilizers that are also present in the vaccine. To make matters worse, the MMR vaccine is often administered at the same time as the Hep B, Hib, IPV (polio), varicella (chickenpox) and PCV (pneumococcal) vaccines. Potentially eight vaccines injected into a 12-month-old infant on the same day.[29]

With an estimated 80 percent MMR vaccination rate, this leaves around 20 percent or 16 million American children unvaccinated against measles, mumps and rubella. From these 16 million children in 2004 there were only 23 recorded cases of childhood measles, 44 cases of mumps and no cases of rubella.[30] There were no fatalities from these cases. The same percentages apply in New Zealand, with 20 percent of children unvaccinated and no outbreaks of measles since 1997, mumps since 1994 or rubella since 1993.[30]

Vaccine rating – MMR Vaccine

****Highest risk category – This is due to the facts that MMR contains a live virus, is a combination multivalent vaccine and is directly associated with causing an immune/inflammatory response in the brain leading to developmental disorders and autistic symptoms.

PCV (PNEUMOCOCCAL CONJUGATE VACCINE)

The *Streptococcus pneumococcal* bacteria are associated with ear infections and, more rarely, pneumonia and meningitis in children. There are a total of 90 different strains of this bacteria, which can typically be found in the ears, noses and throats of many people without any symptoms. The bacteria are spread by sneezing, coughing and exposure to respiratory secretions. When a child's immune system is weakened or vulnerable, contact with this bacteria may lead to an infection.[32]

Pneumococcal bacteria don't appear to pose much of a threat to children with a healthy immune system. They are found in the ears, noses and throats of approximately 50 percent of all young children at any one time, without any symptoms being present.[33] Annually in the U.S., systemic pneumococcal infection is responsible for about 100 deaths in children under 5 years old each year. In England it's responsible for about 35 deaths in children of this age. According to the *American Journal of Public Health*, older age and underlying disease are the most important contributing factors to death from *Pneumococcal pneumonia*, the bacteria that cause pneumonia.[34] When the immune system is working properly, it keeps the *Pneumococcal* bacteria in check and prevents them from causing infection.

The most commonly used Pneumococcal conjugate vaccine (PCV) is Prevnar, which contains parts of the cell membranes of seven different species of the virus. It was first introduced in 2000 and is routinely administered at 2, 4, 6 and 12 months of age. It is available as an individual vaccine, but it is commonly injected at the same time as Hep B, DTaP, Hib and IPV, making it part of the seven vaccines (remember, DTaP is three different vaccines) routinely injected at two-month intervals in a baby's first year of life.

Since this vaccine was first introduced, infections associated with the seven species of *Streptococcus pneumococcus* found in the vaccine have decreased. Unfortunately, infections caused by the other 83 species have steadily *increased*. Between 2000 and 2001, the percentage of pneumococcal ear infections caused by strains not addressed by Prevnar more than doubled from 16 to 37 percent[35], a phenomenon that has been referred to as the "replacement" effect, which means that infection from the other forms of Streptococcus increase as competition from the seven strains in the vaccine decreases.[36] This is exactly the same way that antibiotics have created an ever-increasing number of super-bugs and antibiotic-resistant strains of bacteria. And the longer Prevnar is in use, the more pronounced this effect becomes.

The best protection for your child from all forms of bacteria and viruses is a strong, healthy and fully functioning immune system. Vaccines can modify and create some degree of immunity against a relatively small number of infections. However, when this small spectrum of immunity creates a larger deficiency in overall immune function, the benefit is not worth the cost.

Vaccine rating – Pneumococcal Conjugate Vaccine

**Medium risk category – When given individually, the PCV carries a medium risk of immune and brain dysfunction with an increased chance of developing infection from the other forms of *Streptococcus pneumococcus*. The rating increases to highest risk if PCV is injected at the same time as DTaP, IPV, Hep B and Hib vaccines, because of the accumulative burden and toxic effect created by giving multiple vaccines simultaneously.

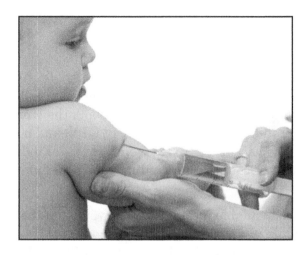

OPV - IPV (POLIO)

Polio infection (*poliomyelitis*) strikes when the polio virus invades the central nervous system and damages motor nerve cells. Depending on which parts of the nervous system are affected, symptoms can include muscle weakness, muscular paralysis and the deformation of limbs. The virus is primarily transmitted via the fecal matter hand-mouth route, and good hygiene and proper sanitation are extremely effective ways to prevent exposure and transmission.

The largest recorded polio outbreak in America occurred in 1952 when 57,628 people contracted the disease. In response to the outbreak, a polio vaccine made from the inactivated polio virus (IPV), was developed by Dr. Jonas Salk and introduced in 1955. Then, in 1961, an oral polio vaccine (OPV) containing live polio virus was introduced. The polio virus for this vaccine was cultured and grown in the laboratory on monkey kidneys that also contained the SV40 virus, and the polio vaccines became contaminated with the SV40 virus. Since then, adults and children who received that particular vaccine have been found to have increased rates of cancer, osteosarcoma and mesothelioma, and the

SV40 virus has been found directly inside the brain tumors, bone cancers, lung cancers and mesotheliomas in those who received this vaccine.[37]

The OPV contaminated with the SV40 virus is documented to have been in use from 1962 to 1999.[38] In 2000, the United States government prohibited any further use of OPV, and now only the inactivated polio vaccine (IPV) is given.[39] However, OPV continues to be used in other countries, including New Zealand.[40]

This vaccine is available individually; however, on the regular vaccine schedule it is usually given at 2 months, 4 months and 15 months of age along with DTaP, Hib, and PCV. This makes a total of six vaccines (DTaP contains three different vaccines) being injected into a 2-month-old baby in one office visit...and then the same six vaccines being injected again just 2 months later.

Nobody can really dispute that the polio vaccine has had a huge impact on the scope of the disease worldwide. However, today, 50 years after the vaccine was introduced, polio is no longer a problem. There have been no cases in the United States since 1991, and no cases in New Zealand since 1961. In fact, America was declared polio-free in 1994[41] and Europe attained the same status in 2002.[42,43] To put the incidence of polio in perspective, lightning kills 100 people and injures another 1,000 in America each year.[44] Your child has a greater chance of being struck by lightning than catching polio.

The live oral polio vaccine (OPV) introduced and used from 1962 to 1999 resulted in an average of 8-10 cases of vaccine-caused poliomyelitis each year.[45] These vaccine-caused cases of polio in America have stopped with the change to the inactivated polio vaccine (IPV). The last case of wild polio (polio contracted without exposure to the vaccination) in America was detected in 1991. The last solitary case of wild polio in New Zealand occurred in 1961.

Since that time, there have been four cases of vaccine-caused poliomyelitis in New Zealand.[46]

There are now only four countries in the world where polio remains a risk: India, Nigeria, Pakistan and Afghanistan. Ninety-nine percent of all the world's polio cases (a total of 2,000 in 2006) are concentrated in just three countries: India, Nigeria and Pakistan.[47]

Vaccine rating - Polio (OPV – live oral polio vaccine)

** Medium risk category – if administered by itself. However, this is elevated to highest risk if OPV vaccine is given in the same office visit with five other vaccines, as with the typical vaccine schedule.

Vaccine rating - Polio (IPV– inactivated polio vaccine)

** Medium risk category – if administered by itself. However, this is elevated to highest risk if IPV vaccine is given in the same office visit with five other vaccines, as with the typical vaccine schedule. This greatly increases the chance of adverse reactions due to accumulative immune burden and toxicity.

VARICELLA (CHICKENPOX)

Chickenpox, which is caused by the varicella-zoster virus, has historically always been considered a normal childhood illness. When contracted in childhood, chickenpox is normally never life threatening, and exposure can help form a strong immune system by developing lifelong antibodies to the chickenpox virus and extra resistance against the associated family of varicella viruses, which includes all of the herpes viruses.

The varicella vaccine, first introduced in 1995, incorporates a live virus but *does not* create lifelong immunity. It is usually injected once at about 12 months of age, with a booster shot at 4-6 years. It is available as an individual vaccine, but is often given to the child at 12 months along with Hep B, Hib, IPV, MMR and PCV. That makes a grand total of eight vaccines in one visit! (MMR is a combination of three vaccines.)

The introduction of this vaccine suddenly changed chickenpox from a normally occurring childhood illness into a reason for one more vaccine to be added to the burden imposed on a child. As with all vaccines, you the parent should make an informed, educated and considered decision regarding the adverse potentials to which you are exposing your child. Does the risk of catching a benign infection like chickenpox, from which generations of children have easily recovered, warrant the risks inherent in taking the vaccine?

Vaccine rating – Varicella

** Medium risk category if given by itself. However, it is usually classified as highest risk category due to its being a live virus vaccine, and because it is almost always given simultaneously with several other vaccines. This creates an accumulative toxic and immune burden, which can then cause an inflammatory/immune reaction in the body and inside the brain.

ROTAVIRUS

Rotavirus is the most common cause of severe diarrhea among

infants and young children, and is one of several viruses that cause infections often called stomach flu, despite having no relation to influenza. By the age of 5, nearly every child in the world has been infected with rotavirus at least once. However, with each infection immunity develops and subsequent infections are less severe. Rotavirus A, the most common form of this virus, causes more than 90 percent of infections in humans.

The virus is transmitted by the fecal-oral route, so sanitation and good hygiene can play a major part in preventing contact or reducing the likelihood of recurrent infection. Rotavirus infection is characterized by vomiting, watery diarrhea, and low-grade fever. Once a child is infected by the virus, there is an incubation period of about two days before symptoms appear. Symptoms often start with vomiting, followed by four to eight days of diarrhea. Rotavirus is usually an easily managed childhood infection with treatment primarily involving management of symptoms and most importantly, the maintenance of hydration.

On May 7th, 2010 the FDA publicly announced the fact that a porcine circovirus (PCV1), a pig virus, had been recently found as a contaminant in GlaxoSmithKline's rotavirus vaccine, and that it had been unknowingly present in the vaccine since it was first developed and introduced in 2008.

The FDA told doctors to immediately stop the use of the Rotarix vaccine for rotavirus immunization due to the contamination of this vaccine with the pig virus.

In the same week, it was also disclosed that another pig virus, potentially an even more dangerous variety called porcine circovirus 2 (PCV2), was found as a contaminant in the other rotavirus vaccine given to children, Merck's RotaTeq vaccine. PCV2 virus causes the following symptoms in infant pigs:

- Wasting and failure to thrive

- Immune suppression

- Respiratory problems

- Kidney, brain and reproductive problems

- Death

Vaccine rating – Rotavirus

**** Highest risk category due to high number of adverse reactions since first introduced and documented history of ongoing contamination with other animal viruses, including aforementioned pig viruses.

Appendix III

Chapter References

Overview

1. Perrin, J, Bloom, S., Gortmaker, S., The Increase of Childhood Chronic Conditions in the United States. *JAMA*, 2007: 297: 2755-2759

2. Polanczyk, G., de Lima, MS, Horta, BL, Biederman, J, Rohde, LA (2007). "The worldwide prevalence of ADHD: a systematic review and metaregression analysis". *Am J Psychiatry* 164 (6): 942–48.

3. E.Isolauri, A. Hurrie, S., The allergy epidemic extends beyond the past few decades. *Clinical Exp. Allergy* 2004, 34 (7): 1007-1110

4. Kamal Elderirawi, MS, Victoria Persky, History of Ear Infections and Prevalence of Asthma in a National Sample of Children aged 2 to 11 years. The Third National Health and Nutrition Examination Survey, 1988 to 1994.

5. Lamphear, BP, Byrd, RS, et al. Increasing prevalence of recurrent otitis media among children in the United States. *Pediatrics* 1997: 99: E1

6. Hedley, AA, Ogden, CL, Johnson, CL, Carroll, Curtin, LR, Flegal, KM. "Overweight and obesity among US children, adolescents,

and adults." 1999-2002. JAMA 291:2847-50. 2004. National Center for Health Statistics.

7.   Muntner, P, He, J, Cutler, J.A., Wildman, R.P., Whelton, P.K. "Trends in Blood Pressure Among Children and Adolescents"*JAMA*. May 5 2004; 291:2107-2113 pg.

8.   Fagot-Campagna, A, Pettitt, DJ, Engelgau, MM, et al. "Type 2 Diabetes among North American children and adolescents: an epidemiologic review and public health perspective." *J. Pediatrics* 2000; 136 (5):664-72.

9.   Asher, M., Montefort, S., Strachan, P., Weiland D., Williams, H., Worldwide time trends in the prevalence of symptoms of asthma, allergic rhinoconjunctivitis, and eczema in childhood: ISAAC Phases One and Three repeat multicountry cross-sectional surveys.*The Lancet* 2006; 368:733-743

10. Fombonne, E. Epidemiological Surveys of Autism and Other Pervasive Developmental Disorders: An Update. *Journal of Autism and Developmental Disorders* 2003;33(4):365-82.

11. Newschaffer et al. The Epidemiology of Autism Spectrum Disorders. Annual Review of Public Health, 2007;28:235-258

12. International Autism Epidemiology Network, IAEN, specific article online at; http://www.worldautismawarenessday.org/atf/cf/%7B2DB64348-B833-4322-837C-8DD9E6DF15EE%7D/IAEN_EpiFAQ_2009.pdf

13. Prevalence of Autistic Spectrum Disorders, Autism and Developmental Disabilities Monitoring Network, United States, 2002, MMWR 2007,56

14. Perrin, James, Bloom, S., Gortmaker S., The Increase of Childhood Chronic Conditions in the United States. *JAMA*, 2007: 297: 2755-2759

Chapter 1

1.   Popkin, BM, Nielsen, SJ. "The sweetening of the world's diet." *Obesity Research* November 2003;11(11):1325-32. Available online at www.obesityresearch.org

2. Duke University, Foundation for Childhood Development, National Center for Health Statistics, Census Bureau, March 31, 2005

3. Hedley, AA, Ogden, CL, Johnson, CL, Carroll,, Curtin, LR, Flegal, KM. "Overweight and obesity among US children, adolescents, and adults." 1999-2002. *JAMA* 291:2847-50. 2004. National Center for Health Statistics.

4. Muntner, P, He, J, Cutler, J.A., Wildman, R.P., Whelton, P.K. "Trends in Blood Pressure Among Children and Adolescents" *JAMA*. May 5 2004; 291:2107-2113 pg

5. Hannon S.T., Goutham R and Arslaninan A.S. "Childhood Obesity and Type 2 Diabetes Mellitus." J Pediatrics, Vol. 116 No. 2 August 2005, pp. 473-480

6. Fagot-Campagna A, Pettitt DJ, Engelgau MM, et al. "Type 2 Diabetes among North American children and adolescents: an epidemiologic review and public health perspective." *J. Pediatrics* 2000; 136 (5):664-72

7. "$67 Million for Anti-Obesity Campaign" New Zealand Harold. Sep 21, 2006. Article available online at http://www.nzherald. co.nz/exercise/news/article.cfm?c_id=500830&objectid=10402329

8. McDonalds Menu Item Details – Available online for all items at http://nutrition.mcdonalds.com/nutritionexchange/itemDetailInfo. do

9. Eastwood J., Vavasour, E. "Safety Evaluation of Certain Food Additives and Contaminants: Diacetyl Tartaric and Fatty Acid Esters of Glycerol." Bureau of Chemical Safety, Food Directorate, Health Products and Food Branch, Health Canada, Ottawa, Ontario, Canada. Available online at http://www.inchem.org/ documents/jecfa/jecmono/v48je02.htm

10. Chen, J. et al. "Safety Evaluation of Certain Food Additives: Evaluation of National Assessments of Intake of Tert-Butylhydroquinone (TBHQ)." World Health Organization. International Programme on Chemical Safety. Chinese Academy of Preventive Medicine, Beijing, China. World Health Organization, Geneva, 1999. IPCS `

11. "GM Foods: A Guide for the Confused." Article available online at

http://www.saynotogmos.org/ud2006/usept06.php#confused

12. United States Department of Agriculture; Guess who is turning 100, "Tracking a century of American eating", Amber Waves, March 2010

13. "Sugar Intake Hits All-time High in 1999." Center for Science in the Public Interest, May 18, 2000, Available online at http://www.cspinet.org/new/sugar_limit.html

14. Jones, W. Borg, S. Boulware, G.,McCarthy, R. "Enhanced adrenomedullary response and increased susceptibility to neuroglycopenia: Mechanisms underlying the adverse effects of sugar ingestion in healthy children." *J Pediatrics*, Volume 126, Issue 2, Pages 171-177 (1995)

15. Benton, D., Maconie, A., et al. (2007). "The influence of the glycaemic load of breakfast on the behaviour of children in school." *Physiol Behav* 92(4): 717-24. Available online at http://www.ncbi.nlm.nih.gov/entrez/query.fcgi?cmd=Retrieve&db=PubMed&dopt=Citation&list_uids=17617427

16. Bellisle, F. et al. "Functional Food Science and Behaviour and psychological functions." *British Journal of Nutrition*, 80: S173 – S193 (1998)

17. "Childhood Obesity Report." International Obesity Task Force. May, 2004. Available online at http://www.iotf.org/media/IOTFmay28.pdf

18. Childhood obesity statistics available online at http://www.cga.ct.gov/2002/olrdata/ph/rpt/2002-R-0529.htm

19. "Search for Diabetes in Youth." Center for Disease Control and Prevention, National Center for Chronic Disease Prevention and Health Promotion, Dec 20, 2005, available online at http://www.cdc.gov/diabetes/pubs/factsheets/search.htm

20. Classen, J.B.: Diabetes epidemic follows hepatitis B immunization program. *New Zealand Medical Journal*, 109: 195, 1996

21. Eberhart, MS, Ogden, C., Engelgau, M., Cadwell, B., Hedley, AA, Saydah, SH (November 19, 2004). "Prevalence of Overweight and Obesity Among Adults with Diagnosed Diabetes — United States, 1988-1994 and 1999-2002." *Morbidity and Mortality Weekly*

Report **53** (45):

22. "Americans spend 90% of their food budgets on processed foods". www.sustainabletable.org/issues/additives

23. "Food Color Facts" Food and Drug Administration, 1993. Available online http://www.cfsan.fda.gov/~lrd/colorfac.html

24. Schossler, E. Strawberry flavor ingredients –Why McDonald's Fries Taste So Good." Fast Food Nation (Houghton-Mifflin, 2001) From *The Atlantic Monthly* "http://www.theatlantic.com/issues/2001/01/schlosser.htm 1-17-01"

25. Henkel, J. "Color additives fact sheet." Food and Drug Administration. Available at "http://www.cfsan.fda.gov/%7Edms/cos-221.html" \t "_blank". Nov. 27, 2005.

26. Sasaki, YF, Kawaguchi, S, Kamaya, A, Ohshita, M, Kabasawa, K, Iwama, K, Taniguchi, K, Tsuda, S. "The comet assay with 8 mouse organs; results with 39 currently used food additives." *Mutation Research* (2002 Aug 26); 519(1-2):103-19.

27. Pesticides in the Diets of Infants and Children, National Research Council, National Academy Press, 1993

28. "How safe is your drinking Water? – Herbicides and Insecticides – Specific Chemicals and Health Effects" History of Walter Filters, 2003 "http://www.historyofwaterfilters.com/herbicides-insecticides-2.html"

29. Dubik, M. "Food Colorings, Preservatives, and "Hyperactivity".

30. "Flavoring Suspected in Illness" By Sonya Geis, *Washington Post* Staff Writer, (May 7, 2007); Page A03, http://www.washingtonpost.com/wpdyn/content/article/2007/05/06/AR2007050601089.html

31. Nutrasweet: Health and Safety Concerns - Testimony before Congress Nov 3, 1987. By Richard J. Wurtman, Director of Clinical Research Center, MIT Aspartame (Nutrasweet) Toxicity Information Center "http://www.holisticmed.com/aspartame/"

32. "The effects of a double blind, placebo controlled, artificial food colorings and benzoate preservative challenge on hyperactivity in a general population sample of preschool children." By "http://www.ncbi.nlm.nih.gov/2004 Jun; 89 (6):506-11.

33. "Gastrointestinal Health and the Child with feeding Problems. Part 1: The Issues." New visions, available online at "http://www. new-vis.com/fym/papers/p-feed16.htm"

34. "Antibiotics Kill Your Body's Good Bacteria" by Dr. Joseph Mercola; available online at "http://www.mercola.com/2003/jun/18/ antibiotics_bacteria.htm"

35. "Consumer Concerns About Hormones in Food" Fact Sheet #37, June 2000; Prepared by Renu Gandhi, Ph.D. BCERF Research Associate and Suzanne M. Snedeker, Ph.D., Research Project Leader, BCERF, article available online at "http://envirocancer. cornell.edu/Factsheet/Diet/fs37.hormones.cfm"

36. "The Issues: Artificial Hormones" by Sustainable Table, available online "http://www.sustainabletable.org/issues/hormones/"

37. "Potential Public Health Impacts Of The Use Of Recombinant Bovine Somatotropin In Dairy Production" September 1997, by Michael Hansen, Ph.D., Jean M. Halloran, Edward Groth III, Ph.D., Lisa Y. Lefferts; prepared for a scientific review by the joint expert committee on Food Additives

38. "EU Scientists Confirm Health Risks of Growth Hormones in Meat." Associated Press April 23, 2002; online "http://www. organicconsumers.org/toxic/hormone042302.cfm"

39. Center for Disease Control and Prevention: "Third National Report on Human Exposure to Environmental Chemicals, Spotlight on Mercury" (1999); available on the United States Environmental Protection Agency website: "http://www.epa.gov/ mercury/effects.htm"

40. "Toxicological Effects of Methylmercury." Committee on the Toxicological Effects of Methylmercury. Board on Environmental Studies and Toxicology. Commission on Life Sciences. National Research Council. National Academy Press, (2000) Washington D.C. Book available online at "http://books.nap.edu/openbook. php?isbn=0309071402"

41. U.S. Environmental Protection Agency: "Health Effects of PCBs (Polychlorinated Biphenyls)" available online "http://www.epa. gov/pcb/pubs/effects.html"

42. Mendola, P. et al, 1997. "Consumption of PCB-contaminated

Freshwater Fish and Shortened Menstrual Cycle Length." *American Journal of Epidemiology*, 145(11): 955.

43. Stewart, P. et al 2000. "Prenatal PCB exposure and neonatal behavioral assessment scale (NBAS) performance." *Neurotoxicology and Teratology*, 22: 21-29.

44. "Dietary Reference Intakes: The Essential Guide to Nutrient Requirements." (September 2006) The National Academy Press, U.S. National Academy of Sciences.

45. D'Adamo, James, Richards, Allan. *One Man's Food is Someone Else's Poison* 1980 Health Thru Herbs Inc. ISBN 0-399-90092-6

46. D'Adamo, Peter, Whitney, Catherine. *Eat Right 4 Your Type – Complete Blood Type Encyclopedia*. Riverhead Books, Penguin Putnam, New York, N.Y. (Jan. 2002) ISBN 1-57322-920-2.

47. D'Adamo, Peter, Whitney, Catherine. *Eat Right 4 Your Type – Complete Blood Type Encyclopedia* Riverhead Trade. The Berkley Publishing Group. New York, NY. (2002) Pg. 343-353.

48. Khader, Dina, Toovey, Irene. *The Food Combining/Blood Type Diet Solution. The Blood Type Theory, Food Lectins*. McGraw-Hill Professionals Publishing. March, 2000. 1 ed. 153:4.

49. McCance, R.A., Widdowson, E.M. "McCance and Widdowson's the Composition on Food: Summary Edition." (6th Edition) The Royal Society of Chemistry (2002) 538 pg.

50. Poongothai, R., Ravikrishnan P., Endocrine Disruption and Perspective Human Health Implications: A Review. *The Internet Journal of Toxicology*. 2008 Volume 4 Number 2.

51. Worthington, V. "Nutritional Quality of Organic Versus Conventional Fruits, Vegetables, and Grains." *The Journal of Alternative Medicine* 2001. Vol 7 (2): 161-173.

52. Worthington, Virginia. "Analyzing Data to Compare Nutrients in Conventional Versus Organic Crops." The *Journal of Alternative and Complementary Medicine*. Oct 2002, Vol. 8, No. 5: 529-532.

53. Steingraber, S. *Living Downstream - An Ecologist looks at Cancer and the Environment*. (1997) New York, Addison - Wesley Publishing Company, Inc.

54. Perrin, J.M., Bloom, S.R., Gortmaker, S. L. "The Increase of Childhood Chronic Conditions in the United States." *JAMA.* (June 27), 2007; Vol. 297:2755-2759.

55. "PCBs in Farmed Salmon. Results from tests of store-bought farmed salmon show seven of 10 fish were so contaminated with PCBs that they raise cancer risk." Environmental Working Group. July, 2003. Available online at http://www.ewg.org/reports/farmedpcbs

56. "US: High pesticide level marks 'Dirty Dozen' fruits, vegetables." Environmental Working Group. October 18, 2006. Article available online at http://www.ewg.org/node/18866

57. Keen, CL., Zidenberg-Cherr, S. "Should vitamin-mineral supplements be recommended for all women with childbearing potential?" *American Journal of Clinical Nutrition.* 1994 Feb; 59(2 Suppl): 532S-538S.

58. Dani, J., Burrill, C., Demmig-Adams, B., "The remarkable role of nutrition in learning and behaviour." *Journal of Nutrition & Food Science*, 2005, Vol 35. 4: (258-263)

59. Helland. B., Smith. L., Saarem. K.,. Saugstad. O., Drevon. C., "Maternal Supplementation With Very-Long-Chain n-3 Fatty Acids During Pregnancy and Lactation Augments Children's IQ at 4 Years of Age" *Pediatrics.*Vol. 111 No. 1 January 2003, pp. e39-e44.

60. Bartlett, J. "Understanding Fats and the Human Brain." Gold Coast Chiropractic Center. Article available online at http://www.jbnat.com/articles/understanding_fats.pdf

61. Helland, B., Smith. B.,,Saarem. K., Saugstad. O., Drevon. C., "Maternal Supplementation With Very-Long-Chain n-3 Fatty Acids During Pregnancy and Lactation Augments Children's IQ at 4 Years of Age" *Pediatrics* Vol. 111 No. 1 January 2003, pp. e39-e44.

62. "Vitamin C History" Available online at http://www.beta-glucan-info.com/vitaminchistory.htm

63. Han, JM, Chang, BJ, Li, TZ, Choe, NH, Quan, FS, Jang, BJ, Cho, IH, Hong, HN, Lee, JH. "Protective effects of ascorbic acid against lead-induced apoptic neurodegeneration in the developing rat

hippocampus in vivo." *Brain Research*. 2007 Dec 14; 1185:68-74.

64. Gorton, HC, Jarvis, K. "The effectiveness of vitamin C in preventing and relieving the symptoms of virus-induced respiratory infections." *J Manipulative Physiol Ther*. 1999;22(8):530-533.

65. Gill, H, Prasad, J. "Probiotics, immunomodulation and health benefits." *Advanced Experiments of Medical Biology*. 2008; 606: 423-54.

66. Winkler, P, de Vrese, M, Laue, Ch, Schrezenmeir, J. "Effect of a dietary supplement containing probiotic bacteria plus vitamins and minerals on common cold infections and cellular immune parameters." *Int J Clin Pharmacol Ther*. 2005 Jul;43(7):318-26.

Chapter 2

1. Branum, A. M., Lukacs, S. L. "Food Allergy Among U.S. Children: Trends in Prevalence and Hospitalization." NCHS Data Brief. Center for Disease Control and Prevention. Department of Health and Human Services. Number 10, October 2008. Article available online at http://www.cdc.gov/nchs/data/databriefs/db10.htm

2. Iannelli, V. "Food Allergies. When Food Becomes and Enemy." Article available online at http://pediatrics.about.com/cs/ conditions/a/food_allergies.htm December,2006.

3. Asero, R. "Multiple intolerance to food additives." *J Allergy Clin Immunol* 2002; 110:531.

4. Sampson, HA. "Update on food allergy." *J Allergy Clin Immunol*; 113:805-19. 2004.

5. Rapp, Doris, M.D. "Can allergies cause behavior problems?" Discussion available online at http://drrapp.blogspot.com/

6. Gershon, Michael, M.D., *The Second Brain: The Groundbreaking New Understanding of Nervous Disorders of the Stomach and Intestine*. Harper Paperbacks (November 17, 1999).

7. Bock, SA., Buckley, J, Holst, A, May, CD. "Proper use of skin tests with food extracts in diagnosis of hypersensitivity to food in

children." *Clin Allergy* 1977; 7(4):375-383.

8. Sampson, HA, Albergo, R. "Comparison of results of skin tests, RAST, and double-blind, placebo-controlled food challenges in children with atopic dermatitis." *J Allergy Clin Immunol* 1984; 74(1):26-33.

Chapter 3

1. Guynup, Sharon. "Toxins Accumulate in Arctic Peoples." National *Geographic*, (Aug 27, 2004) Online at "http://news. nationalgeographic.com/news/2004/08/0827 040827 tvarctic toxins.html"

2. Walton, D., M.D. ed. "British Antarctic Survey - Regional Based Assesment of Persistent Toxic Substances." Antarctica Regional Report. United Nations Environment Programme Chemicals. Global Environment Facility. (Dec. 2002) P. 22-32; 39-50. Online at "http://www.chem.unep.ch/Pts/regreports/Antarctica%20 full%20report.pdf"

3. Landrigan, Philip J., Schechter, Clyde B., Lipton, Jeffrey M., Fahs, Marianne C. and Schwartz, Joel. "Environmental pollutants and disease in American children: estimates of morbidity, mortality, and costs for lead poisoning, asthma, cancer, and developmental disabilities." *Environmental Health Perspectives* (2002) Jul;110(7): 721-8

4. "State of the Air 2005 Report" American Lung Association (2005) Online at http://lungaction.org/reports/sota05_full.html

5. Bubny P., 2006, Eco Protect: Vitamin Retailer, Nov. 37-39.

6. United States Environmental Protection Agency – Toxic Release Inventory Data (TRI) Program. (2007) Online at "http://www. epa.gov/tri/" See also: "Scorecard." The Pollution Information site – online http://www.scorecard.org/env-releases/county.tcl?fips county_code=06037

7. Mount Sinai School of Medicine (New York), Environmental Working Group and Commonweal. "The Body Burden – The Pollution in People." Online at http://www.ewg.org/reports/

bodyburden1/es.php

8.   Yardley, J. (2005) "China's next big boom, could be foul air." *New York Times*, Oct 30, 2003

9.   "Body Burden — The Pollution in Newborns. A benchmark investigation of industrial chemicals, pollutants and pesticides in umbilical cord blood." Environmental Working Group, (July 14, 2005) Online at "http://www.ewg.org/reports/bodyburden2/execsumm.php

10. Massey, Stephen M. "Russia's Maternal & Child Health Crisis: Socio-Economic Implications and the Path Forward." (2002) East West Institute Policy Brief. Vol. 1 No. 9. (10 Dec 2002) Full text available at http://psp.iews.org

11. Wagner, T. *In Our Backyard: A Guide to Understanding Pollution and its Effects* (New York: Van Nostrand Reinhold, 1994) 78

12. The American Lung Association – 2008 Pollution Report. "First city outside California (Pittsburg) Tops one of the Most-Polluted Lists. National Trends Show that Declines in Ozone and Particulate Pollution Have Stalled." Press release available online at http://www.lungusa.org/site/c.dvLUK9O0E/b.34894/apps/s/content.asp?ct=5318243 (May 1, 2008).

13. Environmental Protection Agency "Estimating Exposure to Dioxin-Like Compounds." vols. 1-3, EPA/600/6-88/005Ca,b,c (Washington, D.C.:EPA, 1994); EPA, Health Assessment Document for 2,3,7,8-Tetrachlorodibenzo-p-dioxin (TCDD) and Related Compounds, vols. 1-3, EPA/600/BP-92/001a,,b,c (Washington, D.C.:EPA, 1994)

14. Masayuki, S., Motoaki, A.,. "Effect of outdoor nitrogen dioxide on respiratory symptoms in schoolchildren." *International Journal of Epidemiology*. 2000;29:862-870.

15. Lloyd, A., Cackette, T., (2001) "Diesel Engine: Environmental Impact and Control" California Air Resources Board, Air & Waste Management Association 51:809-847

16. Pope, C.A., III, et al. (2002) "Lung Cancer, cardiopulmonary mortality, and long-term exposure to fine particulate pollution"*JAMA*, 287:1123-1141.

17. Health Effects of Polycyclic Aromatic Hydrocarbons. Source:

Agency for Toxic Substances and Disease Registry. The Encyclopedia of Earth. Online at http://www.eoearth.org/article/ Health_effects_of_Polycyclic_aromatic_hydrocarbons

18. "Lead in Paint, Dust and Soil –Health Effects of Lead." Environmental Protection Agency. Online at http://www.epa.gov/ lead/pubs/leadinfo.htm#facts

19. Sokol, R., Kraft; P., et. al.,. "Exposure to environmental ozone alters semen quality." *Environmental Health Perspectives*. 2006 March; 114(3): 360-365

20. Bertazzi, P.A., Consonni, D., Bachetti, S., Rubagotti, M., Baccarelli, A., Zocchetti. C., Pesatori. A. (2001) "Health Effects of Dioxin Exposure: A 20-Year Mortality Study" *American Journal of Epidemiology* Vol. 153, No. 11 : 1031-1044

21. Kogevinas, M. (2001) "Human health effects of dioxins: cancer, reproductive and endocrine system effects." *Human Reproduction Update,* Vol.7, No.3 pp.331-339.http://humupd.oxfordjournals.org/ misc/terms.shtml

22. Barzilian, J., *The Water We Drink*. Rutgers Univ. Press, 1999

23. Ibid, P.140

24. Ibid P.140

25. "How safe is your drinking Water? – Herbicides and Insecticides – Specific Chemicals and Health Effects" History of Walter Filters, 2003 "http://www.historyofwaterfilters.com/herbicides-insecticides-2.html"

26. Schettler T. Toxic threats to neurologic development of children. *Environ Health Perspect* 2001 Dec;109 Suppl 6:813-6)

27. "Lead in Paint, Dust and Soil –Health Effects of Lead." Environmental Protection Agency. Online at http://www.epa.gov/ lead/pubs/leadinfo.htm#facts

28. *Toxicological Effects of Methylmercury*. Committee on the Toxicological Effects of Methylmercury. Board on Environmental Studies and Toxicology. Commission on Life Sciences. National Research Council. National Academy Press, (2000) Washington D.C. Book available online at "http://books.nap.edu/openbook. php?isbn=0309071402"

29. Center for Disease Control and Prevention: "Third National Report on Human Exposure to Environmental Chemicals, Spotlight on Mercury" (1999); Available on the United States Environmental Protection Agency website: "http://www.epa.gov/mercury/effects.htm"

30. Stewart, P. et al 2000. "Prenatal PCB exposure and neonatal behavioral assessment scale (NBAS) performance." *Neurotoxicology and Teratology*, 22: 21-29.

31. Brouwer, A., Longnecker, M., et al., "Characterization of potential endocrine-related health effects at low-dose levels of exposure to PCBs." *Environmental Health Perspectives*. 1999, 107(Supplement 4): 639–649.

32. U.S. Environmental Protection Agency: "Health Effects of PCBs (Polychlorinated Biphenyls)" available online "http://www.epa.gov/pcb/pubs/effects.html

33. Jacobson, J. L. and Jacobson, S. W. "Intellectual Impairment in Children Exposed to Polychlorinated Biphenyls in Utero." *New England Journal of Medicine*, (1996) 335(11): 783-789.

34. Windham, Gayle C., Lee, Diana, Mitchell, Patrick, Anderson, Meredith, Petreas, Myrto, Lasley, Bill. "Exposure to Organochlorine Compounds and Effects on Ovarian Function." *Epidemiology*. March 2005. Vol 16 (2): 182-190

35. Canfield, RL, et al. "Intellectual impairment in children with blood lead concentrations below 10 µg per deciliter." *New England Journal of Medicine* April 17, 2003; 348:1517-26.

36. Thomson, GO, Raab, GM, Hepburn, WS, Hunter, R, Fulton, M, Laxen, DP. "Blood-lead levels and children's behavior-results from the Edinburgh Lead Study." *Journal of Child Psychology and Psychiatry* 1989; 30:515-528.

37. Needleman, HL, Schell, A, Bellinger, D, Leviton, A, Allred, EN. "The long-term effects of exposure to low doses of lead in childhood. An 11-year follow-up report." *New England Journal of Medicine* 1990; 322:83-8.

38. Royal, Michael A. "Amalgam Fillings: Do Dental Patients Have a Right to Informed Consent?" Pierce Law Center http://www.piercelaw.edu/Risk/Vol2/spring/Royal.htm

39. "Consumer Advisory." U.S. FDA, Food Safety Website, March 2004 http://www.cfsan.fda.gov/~dms/admehg.html

40. "Mercury – Investigation of General Ban. Report by the Swedish Chemicals Inspectorate in response to a Commission from the Swedish Government." Swedish Chemicals Inspectorate. Stockholm, October 2004. Available online at: http://www.kemi.se/upload/Trycksaker/Pdf/Rapporter/Rapport4_04.pdf

41. Gray, LE, Ostby, J, Furr, J, Price, M, Rao, Veeramachaneni DN, Parks, L. "Phthalates and male sexual differentiation." (2000) *Toxicological Sciences* 58, 350-365.

42. Sathyanarayana, S., Karr, C.J., Lozano, P., Brown, E., Calafat, A.M., Liu, F. and Swan, S.H. "Baby care products: Possible sources of Infant Phthalate Exposure." *Pediatrics* Vol 121 No. 2 February 2008, pp. e260-e268.

43. Toxic Softener to be Banned in Europe." Environment News Service. Sept. 28, 2004. Online at http://www.ens-newswire.com/ens/sep2004/2004-09-28-01.asp

44. S. vom Saal, Frederick. Hughes, Claude. "Bisphenol A - An extensive new literature concerning low dose effects of Bisphenol A" *Environmental Health Perspectives.*, 2005 August, 113(8) 926-933

45. Fischer, D., Hooper, K., Athanassiadis, I., and Bergman, A. "Children Show Highest Levels of Polybrominated Diphenyl Ethers in a California Family of Four: A Case Study." *Environmental Health Perspectives.* 2006 114:1581-1584.

46. Adams, A.J. International Institute of Holistic Healing: What is Far Infrared Therapy and How Does it Work Toward Healing the Body? (www.drajadams.com/SaunaDomeInfrared.html)

47. Rogers, M.D., Sherry A.: Detoxify Or Die. Sarasota, FL: Sand Key Company, Inc., pgs. 199-200; 206-13, 2002

Chapter 4

1. Cunha, B., et al. Adverse effects of Antibiotics. *Heart and Lung* 13:5 (1984), 465-472. Gilman, A., et al, Goodman and Gilman's

The Pharmaceutical Basis of Therapeutics. Sixth Edition. New York: Macmillan, 1980, 1148-1150

2. Finch, R., Immunomodulating effects of antimicrobial agents. *J. Antimicrobial Chemotherapy* 6 (1980), 691-699. Gilman, A., et al op.cit., 1224

3. Dowell, S. F., Marcy, M. S., Phillips, W. R., Gerber, M. A., and Schwartz, B., Otitis Media - Principles of Judicious Use of Antimicrobial Agents." *Pediatrics,* Vol. 101 No. 1 Supplement January 1998, pp. 165-171.

4. Wang, E.L., Einarson, T.R., Kellner, J.D., Conly, J.M., "Antibiotic Prescribing for Canadian Preschool Children: Evidence of Over prescribing for Viral Respiratory Infections." Clinical Infectious Diseases. University of Chicago. 1999;29 pg. 155.

5. The list of pharmaceutical drugs' side effects are alphabetically listed on the web under "Drug Side Effects" at http://www.drugs.com/sfx/

6. "Linus Pauling – Biography" available online by the free encyclopedia http://en.wikipedia.org/wiki/Linus_Pauling

7. Frymann, Viola. D.O. "What is Osteopathic Manipulation?" Osteopathic Center for Children and Families. Available online at http://www.osteopathiccenter.org/whatis.html

8. "Chinese Herbology" Comprehensive summary of the fundamental Chinese Herbs online at http://en.wikipedia.org/wiki/Chinese_herbology

9. Haldeman, S., et al. *Principles and Practice of Chiropractic.* Chapter 1: History of Spinal Manipulation by Glenda Wiese and Alana Callender" McGraw-Hill Publishing Company. Pg 624 (5-22). 2nd Ed. 1994

10. Jing, Chen. *Anatomical Atlas of Chinese Acupuncture Points* Shandong Sience and Technology Press, Jinan, China, (1982) 266 pg.

11. Miller, Todd. "Mercury Amalgam Fillings: Human and Environmental Issues Facing the Dental Profession." DePaul Journal of Health Care Law. 1:355 (1996)

12. "Mercury Free and Healthy - The Dental Amalgam Issue." DAMS

Inc. 1079 Summit Ave, Saint Paul, MN 55105 (2005) Online at http://www.amalgam.org/

13. Ekstrand, J, Björkman, L, Edlund, C, Sandborgh-Englund, G. "Toxicological aspects on the release and systemic uptake of mercury from dental amalgam." *European Journal of Oral Sciences*. (1998) Apr: 106 (2 Pt 2):678-86.

14. Neme, AL, Maxson, BB, Linger, JB, Abbott, LJ., "An in-vitro investigation of variables influencing mercury vapor release from dental amalgam." *Operative Dentistry*, 2002 Jan-Feb; 27(1):73-80.

15. Edwards, A. D.D.S. "Thoughts on Biological Dentistry." The International Academy for Biological Dentistry. Article available online at http://www.iabdm.org/ThoughtsBD.html

16. "Mercury vapour in the Oral Cavity – In relation to number of amalgam surfaces/Gold/Porcelain, and the classic symptoms of chronic Mercury Poisoning." Truthful information about dentistry worldwide. The online article is available at http://www.lichtenberg.dk/mercury_vapour_in_the_oral_cavit.htm

17. "Dental Mercury Use Banned in Norway, Sweden and Denmark Because Composites are Adequate..." Reuters Online News service. Article available at http://www.reuters.com/article/pressRelease/idUS108558+03-Jan-2008+PRN20080103

18. "The Clifford Materials Reactivity Testing" Information available online at http://www.ccrlab.com/index.php?option=com_content&task=view&id=19&Itemid=328

Chapter 5

1. "The History of Vaccination" World Health Organization. Online at http://www.childrensvaccine.org/files/WHO-Vaccine-History.pdf

2. Classen, Barthelow, J. "Childhood Immunization and Diabetes Mellitus." *New Zealand, M.J.*, 109, (May 24, 1996), 195.

3. Bradstreet, J., Geier, D.A., Kartzinel, J.J., Adams, J.B., Geier, M.R. "A Case-Control Study of Mercury Burden in Children with Autistic Spectrum Disorders." *Journal of American Physicians and Surgeons*. Vol. 8. No. 3 (2003) pp. 76-79.

4. Geier, Mark R., Geier, David A. "Thimerosal in Childhood Vaccines, Neurodevelopmental Disorders, and Heart Disease in the United States." *Journal of American Physicians and Surgeons.* Vol. 8. No. 1(2003) pp 6-11.

5. Vautier, G., Carty, J.E., "Acute Sero-positive Rheumatoid Arthritis Occurring after Hepatitis Vaccination." *Rheumatology,* 1994. 33:991.

6. Cox, NH, Forsyth, A. "Thimerosal allergy and vaccination reactions." *Contact Dermatitis* (1988) 18:229-233.

7. Rousseau, MC., Parent, ME., St-Pierre, Y. "Potential health effects from non-specific stimulation of the immune function in early age: The example of BCG vaccination." *Pediatrics and Allergy Immunology.* 2007. Dec 21.

8. "Germ theory of disease" Louis Pasteur online at http://en.wikipedia.org/wiki/Germ_theory_of_disease

9. Bechamp, A. "The Blood and Its Third Element." (1867) Available online at http://www.bechamp.org/ official website in the honor of Professor Antoine Bechamp.

10. "The History of Vaccination" World Health Organization. Online at http://www.childrensvaccine.org/files/WHO-Vaccine-History.pdf

11. "A Vaccine Timeline." National Vaccination Information Center. Online at http://www.nvic.org/Timeline/timeline.htm

12. "How Are Vaccines Made" – Vaccine Education Center. Available online at http://www.chop.edu/consumer/jsp/division/generic.jsp?id=75749

13. "SV40 stands for Simian Virus 40." SV40 Cancer Foundation. Available online at http://www.sv40foundation.org/

14. "FDA mishandled Chiron vaccine problems, congressman says" Center For Infectious Disease Research & Policy. Available online at http://www.cidrap.umn.edu/cidrap/content/influenza/general/news/nov2304fda.html

15. "Childhood vaccine is recalled over contamination risks." Source: Associated Press. *Los Angeles Times,* The Nation section (A17). December 13, 2007

16. "Nanobacteria – The New Thing in Heart Disease." Online at http://www.chelationtherapyonline.com/articles/p54.htm

17. "Nanobacteria – The New Thing in Heart Disease." Online at http://www.chelationtherapyonline.com/articles/p54.htm

18. Kinsbourne, Marcel, M.D. "Presentation to the Committee on Government Reform Topic: Vaccines: Finding a Balance between Public Safety and Personal Choice" August 3, 1999 Article available online at http://www.whale.to/vaccines/kinsbourne.html

19. "Thiomerosal" Wikipedia. Available online at http://en.wikipedia.org/wiki/Thiomersal See also, "Thimerosal in Vaccines." U.S. Food and Drug Administration, online at http://www.fda.gov/cber/vaccine/thimerosal.htm

20. "Thimerosal in Seasonal Influenza Vaccine" Center for Disease Control and Prevention. Online at http://www.cdc.gov/flu/about/qa/thimerosal.htm

21. "Vaccine Excipient & Media Summary. Part 2." Center for Disease Control and Prevention. Online at http://www.cdc.gov/vaccines/pubs/pinkbook/downloads/appendices/B/excipient-table-2.pdf

22. "Juvenile Diabetes and Vaccination: New Evidence for a Connection." National Vaccine Information Center. Online at http://www.nvic.org/Diseases/juvenilediabetes.htm

23. National Vaccine Injury Compensation Program (VICP) U.S. department of Health and Services. Online at http://www.hrsa.gov/vaccinecompensation/

24. "History of Pediatric Immunizations." Medscape Free Online Health Database. Available online at http://www.medscape.com/viewarticle/472398_3

25. Perrin, James, M.D., Bloom, S. M.S., Gortmaker .S.. PhD, The Increase of Childhood Chronic Conditions in the United States. *JAMA*, 2007: 297: 2755-2759

26. Lenrot, Roshel K., Giedd, Jay N. "Volumetrics of Brain Development." National Institute of Mental Health, Bethesda, M.D. http://afni.nih.gov/sscc/staff/rwcox/ISMRM_2006/Syllabus percent202006 percent20- percent203340/files/M_06.pdf

27. Blaylock, Russell, M.D. "The Danger of Overvaccination with the Present Vaccine Policy. The Brain's Special Immune System." March 2007. National Health Federation. Online at http://www.thenhf.com/vaccinations_125.htm

28. Blaylock, Russell L., M.D., "Interaction of Cytokines. Excitotoxins. and Reactive Nitrogen and Oxygen Species in Autism Spectrum Disorders" *Journal of the American Nutraceutical Association* Vol.6. No.4 Fall 2003.

29. "FDA Vaccine Testimony" Statement of William Egan, Ph.D. U.S. Food and Drug Administration, September 8, 2004, Available online http://www.autismcoach.com/FDA%20Immunization%20Testimony.htm

Chapter 6

1. Canfield, RL, et al. "Intellectual impairment in children with blood lead concentrations below 10 µg per deciliter." *New England Journal of Medicine* April 17, 2003; 348:1517-26.

2. "The Environmental Outlook in Russia." National Intelligence Council. National Intelligence Estimate. January 1999. Available online at http://www.dni.gov/nic/special_russianoutlook.html

3. Landrigan, P.J., et al. 1998. Children's health and the environment: A new agenda for prevention research. Environmental Health Perspectives 106, Supplement 3:787-794.

4. "Body Burden Community Monitoring Handbook." (2005) The research document is available online at http://www.oztoxics.org/cmwg/bb_introduction.html

5. A Tsiaras, A. Doubleday. *From Conception to Birth - A Life Unfolds.* N.Y. 2002, P8-10 ISBN 0-385-50318-0

6. Ibid pg.

7. Reckeweg, Hains-Heinrich, M.D. "The Adverse Influence of Pork Consumption on Health" Biological Therapy Vol.1 No.2 (1983)

8. "Consumer Advisory." U.S FDA, Food Safety Website, March 2004 http://www.cfsan.fda.gov/~dms/admehg.html

9. McKay, B., Verbeek, M., Jackson, E., Simmonds, M., Landman, J. et al. "Report on the World's Oceans." Greenpeace publication. Greenpeace Research Laboratories Report. May 1998. Available online at http://www.greenpeace.to/publications/reportworldsoceans.pdf

10. "Status and Trends of Fecal Coliform in Shellfish," Washington State Dept of Health, Puget Sound Research, 2001 http://www.psat.wa.gov/Publications/01_proceedings/sessions/oral/1c_deter.pdf

11. King, H.H., Tettambel, M.A., Lockwood, M.D., Johnson, K.H., Arsenault, D.A., Quist, R. "Osteopathic Manipulative Treatment in Prenatal Care: A Retrospective Case Control Design Study." *JAOA*. Vol 103. No. 12. December 2003.

Chapter 7

1. Regenstein, JM. "Health aspects of kosher foods. Activities report and minutes of work groups of the R & D Associates." (1994) 46(1):77-83

2. Reckeweg, Hains-Heinrich, M.D. "The Adverse Influence of Pork Consumption on Health" *Biological Therapy* Vol.1 No.2 (1983)

3. "Status and Trends of Fecal Coliform in Shellfish," Washington State Dept of Health, Puget Sound Research, 2001 http://www.psat.wa.gov/Publications/01_proceedings/sessions/oral/1c_deter.pdf

4. "What You Need to Know About Mercury in Fish and Shellfish." U.S. Food and Drug Administration. 2004 EPA and FDA Advice For: Women Who Might Become Pregnant, Women Who are Pregnant, Nursing Mothers and Young Children. Available online at http://www.fda.gov/Food/FoodSafety/Product-SpecificInformation/Seafood/FoodbornePathogensContaminants/Methylmercury/ucm115662.htm

5. "EWG Tuna Calculator. How much Tuna can you eat Safely? EWG tells you what the FDA won't." Environmental Working Group. January 2004. Available online at http://www.ewg.org/tunacalculator

6. Nettleton Joyce, Seafood: Weighing the Benefits and Risks, Biol Trace Elem Res 2007;119:242-254. *January 2008*.

7. Glenville, M. "Nutritional supplements in pregnancy: commercial push or evidence based?" Current Opinion in Obstetrics and Gynecology 2006 Dec; 18(6): 642-7.

8. Vahratian, A., Siega-Riz, AM., Savitz, DA., Thorp, JM Jr., "Multivitamin use and the risk of preterm birth." *American Journal of Epidemiology* 2004 Nov 1; 160 (9): 886-92.

9. Koren, G. et al. "Study: Prenatal multivitamins prevent wide range of serious birth defects." *Journal of Obstetrics and Gynecology of Canada*. Ottawa. Aug 30, 2006. Available online at http://www.sogc.org/media/pdf/advisories/birth-defect-study-release-aug2006_e.pdf

10. Williamson, R. "Prevention of birth defects: folic acid." *Biology Research in Nursing*. 2001 Jul; 3 (1): 33-8.

11. Zagré, NM., Desplats, G., Adou, P., Mamadoultaibou, A., Aguayo, VM. "Prenatal multiple micronutrient supplementation has greater impact on birthweight than supplementation with iron and folic acid: a cluster-randomized, double-blind, controlled programmatic study in rural Niger." Food Nutrition Bulletin 2007 Sept; 28(3): 317-27.

12. Lira, PI., Ashworth, A., Morris, SS. "Effect of zinc supplementation on the morbidity, immune function, and growth of low birth-weight, full-term infants in northeast Brazil." *The American Journal of Clinical Nutrition*. Vol. 68, pg. 418-424. (1998)

13. Calder, P.C., Kew, S. "The immune system: a target for functional foods?" *British Journal of Nutrition* (2002) 88:S165-S176.

14. Holman, RT, Johnson, SB and Ogburn, PL. "Deficiency of Essential Fatty Acids and Membrane Fluidity During Pregnancy and Lactation." *National Academy of Sciences*, 1991, Vol 88, 4835-4839.

15. Hibbeln, JR. "Seafood consumption, the DHA content of mothers' milk and prevalence rates of postpartum depression: a cross-national, ecological analysis." *Journal of Affective Disorders*. 2002 May;69 (1-3):15-29.

16. Gallagher, S. "Omega 3 oils in pregnancy." *Midwifery Today,* International Midwife. 2004 Spring; (69): 26-31.

17. Helland, I, Smith, L, Saarem, K,. Saugstad, O,. Drevon, C., "Maternal Supplementation With Very-Long-Chain n-3 Fatty Acids During Pregnancy and Lactation Augments Children's IQ at 4 Years of Age" *Pediatrics* Vol. 111 No. 1 January 2003, pp. e39-e44

18. Hoymeyr, GJ, Atallah, AN, Duley, L, "Calcium supplementation during pregnancy for preventing hypertensive disorders and related problems." Cochrane Database System Review. 2006 July 19; 3: CD001059.

19. Ehrenberg, A. "Non-medical prevention of pre-eclampsia." Acta Obstetricia et   Gynecologica Scandinavica. 1997; 164:108-10.

20. Lee, BE, Hong, YC, Lee, KH, Kim, YJ, Kim, WK, Chang, NS, Park, EA, Park, HS, Hann, HJ, "Influence of maternal serum levels of vitamin C and E during the second trimester on birth weight and length." *European Journal of Clinical Nutrition.* 2004 Oct; 58 (10): 1365-71.

21. Hong, J, Park, EA, Kim, YJ, Lee, HY, Park, BH, Ha, EH, Kong, KA, Park, H. "Association of antioxidant vitamins and oxidative stress levels in pregnancy with infant growth during the first year of life." Public Health Nutrition 2007 Dec 7:1-8

22. Han, JM, Chang, BJ, Li, TZ, Choe, NH, Quan, FS, Jang, BJ, Cho, IH, Hong, HN, Lee, JH. "Protective effects of ascorbic acid against lead-induced apoptic neurodegeneration in the developing rat hippocampus in vivo." Brain Research. 2007 Dec 14; 1185:68-74.

23. Douglas, LC, Sanders, ME. "Probiotics and prebiotics in dietetics practice." *Journal of American Dietetics Association.* 2008 March; 108 (3): 510-21.

24. Rodriguez, M, et al.,. "Functional Nutrition and Optimal Nutrition. Near or far?" Servicio de Endocrinología y Nutrición, Hospital Universitario de Getafe, Carretera de Toledo, KM 12,500, 28095 Getafe, Madrid. Rev Esp Salud Publica. 2003 May-June; 77 (3): 317-331. Kopp, MV, Goldstein, M, Dietschek, A, Sofke, J, Heinzmann, A, Urbanek, R. "Lactobacillus GG has in vitro effects on enhanced interleukin-10 and interferon-gamma release of mononuclear cells but no in vivo effects in

supplemented mothers and their neonates." *Clinical Experiment of Allergy*. 2007 Dec 20

25. Rinne, M, Kalliomaki, M, Arvilommi, H, Salminen, S, Isolauri, E. "Effect if probiotics and breastfeeding on the bifidobacterium and lactobacillus/enterococcus microbiota and humoral immune responses." *Journal of Pediatrics*. 2005 Aug; 147 (2): 186-91.

26. Abrahamsson, TR, Jakobsson, T, Böttcher, MF, Fredrikson, M, Jenmalm, MC, Björkstén, B, Oldaeus, G. "Probiotics in prevention of IgE-associated eczema: a double-blind, randomized, placebo-controlled trial." *Journal of Allergy and Clinical Immunology*. 2007 May; 119 (5): 1174-80.

27. Shultz, M, Göttl, C, Young, RJ, Iwen, P, Vanderhoof, JA. "Administration of oral probiotic bacteria to pregnant women causes temporary infantile colonization." *Journal of Pediatrics and Gastroenterology Nutrition*. 2004 March; 38 (3):293-7.

28. Gill, H, Prasad, J. "Probiotics, immunomodulation and health benefits." *Advanced Experiments of Medical Biology*. 2008; 606: 423-54.

29. Kaplas, N, Isolauri, E, Lampi, AM, Ojala, T, Laitinen, K. "Dietary Counseling and probiotic supplementation during pregnancy modify placental phospholipids fatty acids." Lipids. 2007 Sept; 42 (9): 865-70.

30. Jarksi, RW., Trippett, DL., "The risks and benefits of exercise during pregnancy." *The Journal of Family Practice*. 1990 Feb;30(2):185-9.

31. Suputtitada, A. Wacharapreechanont, T., Chaisayan, P. "Effect of the "sitting pelvic tilt exercise" during the third trimester in primigravidas on back pain." *Journal of the Medical Association of Thailand*. 2002 Jun;85 Suppl 1:S170-9.

32. Clap, JF. 3ed. "The course of labor after endurance exercise during pregnancy." *American Journal of Obstetrics and Gynecology*. December, 1990. 163 (6 Pt 1):1799-805.

33. Sternfeld, B., Quesenberry, C.P. Jr., Eskenazi, B., and Newman, L.A. "Exercise during pregnancy and pregnancy outcome." *Clinical Sciences. Medicine & Science in Sports & Exercise*. 27(5):634-640, May 1995

34. Polman, R., Kaiseler, M, Borkoles, E. "Effect of a single bout of exercise on the mood of pregnant women." *The Journal of Sports Medicine and Physical Fitness.* 2007 Mar; 47(1):103-11.

35. Katz, VL. "Water exercise in Pregnancy." Seminars in Perinatololgy. 1996 Aug; 20(4):285-91.

36. Kegel and Tailor exercises can be found online at the University of Michigan, "Smart Moms" website. For more information visit: http://www.med.umich.edu/obgyn/smartmoms/pregnancy/exercise/index.htm

37. Mount Sinai School of Medicine (New York), Environmental Working Group and Commonweal. "The Body Burden – The Pollution in People." Online at http://www.ewg.org/reports/bodyburden1/es.php

38. Wagner, T. *In Our Backyard: A Guide to Understanding Pollution and its Effects* (New York: Van Nostrand Reinhold, 1994) 78

39. Luna, VA, Cannons, AC, Amuso, PT, Cattani, J. "The inactivation and removal of airborne Bacillus atrophaeus endospores from air circulation systems using UVC and HEPA filters." *Journal of Applied Microbiology.* 2008 Feb; 104(2):489-98.

40. "HEPA" Detailed information and description of the high-efficiency particular air (HEPA) filter can be found online at http://en.wikipedia.org/wiki/HEPA

41. King, H.H., Tettambel, M.A., Lockwood, M.D., Johnson, K.H., Arsenault, D.A., Quist, R. "Osteopathic Manipulative Treatment in Prenatal Care: A Retrospective Case Control Design Study." *Journal of the American Osteopathic Association.* December 2003, Vol 103, No 12. pg. 577-582.

42. Gaffney, L., Smith, C., "Use of complementary therapies in pregnancy: The perceptions of obstetricians and midwives in South Australia" Department of Obstetrics and Gynaecology, The University of Adelaide, South Australia, Australia (2003)

43. Hahnemann, Samuel. *Organon of Medicine* Translated by William Boericke M.D. Homeopathic Publications. 15/40- A, Tilak Nagar, New Delhi, India. (1901) 292 pg

44. Smith, CA, Crowther, CA. "Acupuncture for induction of labor." Cochrane Database System Rev 2002;2:CD002962

45. Lennox, D., Betts, S. "Acupuncture for Pre Birth Treatment." *Medical Acupuncture Journal*, 17 (3) May 2006

46. Tenore, J., M.D. "Methods for Cervical Ripening and Induction of Labor" American Family Physician, *Journal of the American Academy of Family Physicians*. (May 15, 2003) Vol. 67/No. 10

47. Parsons, M., "Raspberry Leaf and its effect on labor, safety and efficacy." *Australian College of Midwives Journal*, 12(3) 20-5 Sept. 1999

48. Adair, CD. "Non-pharmacologic approaches to cervical priming and labor induction." *Clinical Obstetrics and Gynecology* (2000) 43:447-54.

49. Moskowitz, R. *Homeopathic Medicines for Pregnancy and Childbirth* (1993) North Atlantic Books Pg. 29-30

50. "Recommended Childhood and Adolescent Immunization Schedule." (2006) Center For Disease Control and Prevention, Department of Health and Human Services. Available online http://www.immunize.org/cdc/child-schedule.pdf

51. Davies, E. "Osteopathy in Pregnancy and Childbirth: A guide for parents and parents-to-be." Available online at http://www.edavies.co.uk/leaflet2.html

52. Frymann, V. "Birth Trauma: The Most Common Cause of Developmental Delays" Osteopathic Center for Children and Families

53. Moskowitz, R. *Homeopathuc Medicines for Pregnancy & Childbirth*. (1993) North Atlantic Books , p. 235

Chapter 8

1. Lenrot, Roshel K., Giedd, Jay N. "Volumetrics of Brain Development." National Institute of Mental Health, Bethesda, M.D. http://afni.nih.gov/sscc/staff/rwcox/ISMRM_2006/Syllabus%202006%20-%203340/files/M_06.pdf

2. Helland, I., et al. "Maternal supplementation with Omega 3 fatty acids during pregnancy and lactation augments children's IQ at 4

years of age." *Journal of Pediatrics* 111(1) 39-44, Jan. 2003.

3.   Makrides, Maria, PhD., Neumann, Mark, A., Simmer, Karen, and Gibson, Robert, A. "A Critical Appraisal of the Role of Dietary Long-Chain Polyunsaturated Fatty Acids on Neural Indices of Term Infants: A Randomized, Controlled Trial." *Pediatrics* Vol. 105 No. 1 January 2000, pp. 32-38

4.   Ouwehand, A., Isolauri, E., Salminen, S. "The role of the intestinal microflora for the development of the immune system in early childhood." *European J. Nutr. [Supp.* 1, (2002): 1/32 – 1/37.

5.   Divi, R., et al. "Anti-thyroid isoflavones from soybean; isolation, characterisation, and mechanisms of action." *Biochemical Pharmacology*, USA 54:1087-96, (1997).

6.   "Soy Infant Formula - Birth Control Pills for Babies. Phytoestrogens in Diets of Infants and Adults" The Weston A. Price Foundation (October 2002) Available online http://www. westonaprice.org/soy/birthcontrolbabies.html

7.   Tuohy, PG. "Soy infant formula and phytoestrogens." *Journal of Paediatrics and Child Health* (August 2003) Volume 39, Issue 6, 401–405

8.   New Zealand Ministry of Health, Position statement: Soy-based Infant Formula, December 1998. Available online http://www. soyonlineservice.co.nz/downloads/mohsoy.pdf

9.   Common Food Allergens. List available online on the official website of The Food Allergy and Anaphylaxis Network at http:// www.foodallergy.org/allergens/index.html

10.   "Forbidden Baby Foods to Avoid" Online article available at http://www.wholesomebabyfood.com/forbiddenbabyfood.htm

11.   Skinner, JD, Carruth, BR, Wendy, B, Ziegler, PJ. "Children's Food Preferences: a longitudinal analysis." *Journal of the American Dietetic Association*, November 2002, Vol. 102 (11); 1638-4.

12.   Fox, MK, Pac, S, Devaney, B, Jankowski, L. "Feeding infants and toddlers study: What foods are infants and toddlers eating?" *Journal of the American Dietetic Association.* January 2002, Vol. 104(1 Supplement 1):s22-30

13. "Prevalence of excess body weight and obesity in children and adolescents." World Health Organization with the collaboration of the European Environment and Health Information System. May 2007, Fact Sheet No. 2.3, Code: RPG2_Hous_E2. Online http://www.euro.who.int/Document/EHI/ENHIS_Factsheet_2_3.pdf

14. Wang, Y., Monteiro, C., Popkin, B. "Trends of obesity and underweight in older children and adolescents in the United States, Brazil, China, and Russia." *American Journal of Clinical Nutrition*, Vol. 75, No. 6, 971-977, June 200

15. Hedley, AA, Ogden, CL, Johnson, CL, Carroll, M.D., Curtin, LR, Flegal, KM. "Overweight and obesity among US children, adolescents, and adults." 1999-2002. *JAMA* 291:2847-50. 2004.

Chapter 9

1. Squires, S. "The Lean Plate - Eat right and your kids are likely to follow." *Los Angeles Times*, Health Section, May 2006

2. Perry, C.L., Klepp, K.I., Dudovitz, B., Golden, D., Griffin, G. and Smyth, M. "Promoting healthy eating and physical activity patterns among adolescents: A pilot study of 'Slice of Life.'" University of Minnesota Division of Epidemiology, School of Public Health 611 Beacon Street SE, Minneapolis, MN 55455, USA Health Education Research, Vol. 2, No. 2, 93-103, 1987.

3. Lindberg, Fedon A. *The Greek Doctor's Diet. A Simple, Delicious, Slow-carb, Mediterranean Approach to Eating and Exercise Designed to Keep You Naturally Slim and Help You to Avoid: Diabetes, Heart Disease, Insulin Resistance, Syndrome X.* Rodale International Ltd. Publishing. London. 2005. pg. 59.

4. Schoenthaler, S. J., Bier, I. D., Young, K., Nichols, D., Jansenns, S. "The Effect of Vitamin-Mineral Supplementation on the Intelligence of American Schoolchildren: A Randomized, Double-Blind Placebo-Controlled Trial." *The Journal of Alternative and Complementary Medicine.* February 2000, 6(1): 19-29.

5. Helland, B, et al., "Maternal Supplementation with Very-Long-Chain n-3 Fatty Acids during Pregnancy and Lactation Augments Children's IQ at 4 Years of Age" *Pediatrics* Vol. 111 No. 1 January

2003, pp. e39-e44.

6. Gorton, HC, Jarvis, K. "The effectiveness of vitamin C in preventing and relieving the symptoms of virus-induced respiratory infections." *J Manipulative Physiol Ther.* 1999; 22 (8):530-533.

7. Chiang, BL., Sheih, YH., Wang, LH., Liao, CK., Gill, HS. "Enhancing immunity by dietary consumption of a probiotic lactic acid bacterium (Bifidobacterium lactis HN019): optimization and definition of cellular immune responses." *European Journal of Clinical Nutrition* (2000) 54, 849-855.

8. McDougall, C. *Born to Run: A Hidden Tribe, Superathletes, and the Greatest Race the World Has Ever Seen.* Random House Publishing. Borzoi Book by Alfred A. Knopf. May 7, 2009.

9. "Diabetes and Obesity Epidemic in Children: International Call to Action." International Diabetes Federation. Press Release, Brussels 2004. Article available online at http://www.diabetes.org. nz/news/world_news/diabetes_and_obesity_epidemic_in_children_ international_call_to_action

10. Grundy, S.M. et al. "Guide to Primary Prevention of Cardiovascular Diseases, A Statement for Healthcare Professionals From the Task Force on Risk Reduction." American Heart Association. 1997. Circulation 95:2329-2331. Available online at http://circ.ahajournals.org/cgi/content/short/95/9/2329

Appendix I

1. Perrin, J.M., Bloom, S.R., Gortmaker, S. L. "The Increase of Childhood Chronic Conditions in the United States." *Journal of the American Medical Association.* (June 27), 2007; Vol. 297:2755-2759.

2. "Asthma Medications Chart" December, 2007, American Lung Association. Available online at http://www.lungusa.org/site/c. dvLUK9O0E/b.263990/

3. D'Adamo, Peter, Whitney, Catherine. *Eat Right 4 Your Type - Complete Blood type Encyclopedia* Riverhead Trade. The Berkley

Publishing Group. New York, NY. (2002) Pg. 343-353.

4. Roxas, M, Jurenka, J. "Colds and influenza: a review of diagnosis and conventional, botanical, and nutritional considerations." *Altern Med Rev.* 2007 Mar;12(1):25-48

5. Warren, MD, Pont, SJ, Barkin, SL, Callahan, ST, Caples, TL, Carroll, KN, Plemmons, GS, Swan, RR, Cooper, WO. "The effect of honey on nocturnal cough and sleep quality for children and their parents." *Arch Pediatr Adolesc Med.* 2007 Dec;161(12):1149-53.

6. Rinne, M, Kalliomaki, M, Arvilommi, H, Salminen, S, Isolauri, E. "Effect if probiotics and breastfeeding on the bifidobacterium and lactobacillus/enterococcus microbiota and humoral immune responses." *Journal of Pediatrics.* 2005 Aug; 147 (2): 186-91.

7. Gill, H, Prasad, J. "Probiotics, immunomodulation, and health benefits." *Advances in Experimental Medicine and Biology.* 2008;606:423-54.

8. Stevenson, LM, Matthias, A, Banbury, L, Penman, KG, Bone, KM, Leach, DL, Lehmann, RP. "Modulation of macrophage immune responses by Echinacea." *Molecules.* 2005 Oct 31;10 (10):1279-85.

9. Hofeldt, FD. Reactive hypoglycemia. *Metabolism* 1975;24:1193–208

10. Anderson, RA et al. "Chromium supplementation of humans with hypoglycemia." *Fed Proc* 1984;43:471

11. Stebbing, JB et al. "Reactive hypoglycemia and magnesium." *Magnesium Bull* 1982;2:131–4.

12. Shansky, A. "Vitamin B3 in the alleviation of hypoglycemia." *Drug Cosm Ind* 1981;129(4):68–69,104

13. Stene, L.C., Ulriksen, J., Magnus, P., and Joner, G.. "Use of cod liver oil during pregnancy associated with lower risk of Type I diabetes in the offspring." *Diabetologia.* Volume 43, No.9: 1093-98. , September, 2000

14. Correa, A., Botto, L., Liu, Y., Mulinare, J. and Erickson, J. D. "Do Multivitamin Supplements Attenuate the Risk for Diabetes-Associated Birth Defects?" *Pediatrics.* Vol. 111 No. 5 May 2003,

pp. 1146-1151

15. "Mullein – Verbascum thapsus" Detailed information and description of this herb can be found online at http://www. altnature.com/gallery/mullien.htm

16. Schoop, R, Klein, P, Suter, A, Johnston, SL. "Echinacea in the prevention of induced rhinovirus colds: a meta-analysis." *Clinical Therapy.* 2006 Feb;28 (2):174-83

Appendix II

1. "Hepatitis B Vaccine Reaction Reports Outnumber Reported Disease Cases in Children According to Vaccine Safety Group." Press Release. National Vaccine Information Center. January 27, 1999. Available online at http://www.nvic.org/nvic-archives/ pressrelease/pressreleasejan271999.aspx

2. Perrin, James, Bloom, S. Gortmaker, S., "The Increase of Childhood Chronic Conditions in the United States" *JAMA*, 2007: 297: 2755-2759

3. "Fatal Respiratory Diphtheria in a U.S. Traveler to Haiti – Pennsylvania, 2003" Center for Disease Control and Prevention. MMWR Newsletter, January 9, 2004 / 52(53);1285-1286. Online at http://www.cdc.gov/mmwr/preview/mmwrhtml/mm5253a3.htm

4. "Vaccines & Immunization – Statistics and Surveillance: Immunization Coverage in the U.S." Center for Disease Control and Prevention. (2006) Coverage available online at http://www. cdc.gov/vaccines/stats-surv/imz-coverage.htm#chart

5. "Child Health USA – 2000-2006 – Vaccine Preventable Diseases." U.S Department of Health and Human Services. Maternal and Child Health Bureau. Available online at http://mchb.hrsa.gov/ chusa02/main_pages/page_02.htm

6. Korobeinikov, A. Maini, P. K. and Walker, W. J. "Estimation of effective vaccination rate: pertussis in New Zealand as a case study." *Journal of Theoretical Biology.* Volume 224, Issue 2, 21 September 2003, Pages 269-275

7. Barkin, R.M., and Pichichero, M.E. "Diphtheria-pertussis-tetanus

vaccine: Reactogenicity of commercial products." (1979) *Pediatrics* 63(2): 256-60.

8. Coulter, Harris L., Fisher Loe, Barbara. *A Shot in the Dark – Why the P in the DPT Vaccination May be Hazardous to Your Children.* Penguin Group Inc. (1991). 246 pg.

9. Durmisević, S, Durmisevict-Serdarević, J. "Side effects of cellular and acellular DPT vaccine in children aged from 3 months to 5 years." Med Pregl. 2004 Nov-Dec; 57(11-12):584-7

10. "2006-07 Influenza (Flu) Season – Questions & Answers" Centers for Disease Control and Prevention. Flu Seasons Summary. Flu Deaths in Children. Available online at http://www.cdc.gov/flu/about/qa/0607season.htm

11. "Influenza Weekly Update – 2007 Reports" Public Health Surveillance. Information for New Zealand Public Health Action. Website available at http://www.surv.esr.cri.nz/virology/influenza_weekly_update.php

12. "Influenza Season in 2007 for Australia and New Zealand" Influenza News November 2007. Influenza Centre. Online at http://www.influenzacentre.org/flunews.htm

13. "Thimerosal in Vaccines – Recent and Future FDA Actions." U.S. Food and Drug Administration. Center for Biologics Evaluation and Research. Available online at http://www.fda.gov/cber/vaccine/thimerosal.htm#tox

14. McCann, T.M. "The use of Homeopathy in the 1921 Flu Epidemic." *The Journal of the American Institute of Homeopathy.* 1921. Reference could be found in a research article, "Some history of the treatment of epidemics with Homeopathy by Julian Winston" online at http://www.whale.to/v/winston.html

15. "Hepatitis, Viral, Type A – Clinical Presentation" Centers for Disease Control and Prevention, Health Information for International Travel 2008, Chapter 4 – Prevention of Specific Infectious Diseases. Online at http://wwwn.cdc.gov/travel/yellowBookCh4-HepA.aspx

16. Wasley, A., Samandari, T., Bell, P., "Incidence of Hepatitis A in the United States in the Era of Vaccination." *The Journal of the American Medical Association.* 2005; 294:194-201.

17. "New Zealand Immunization Schedule – 2008" New Zealand Ministry of Health. Available online at http://www.moh.govt.nz/ moh.nsf/f872666357c511eb4c25666d000c8888/9befb36798f2118ec c256d1e001a5f99?OpenDocument

18. "Australian Standard Vaccination Schedule commencing 2005" Department of Health. Government of Australia. Chart available online at http://www.health.sa.gov.au/PEHS/Immunisation/aust-vacc-schedule-web.pdf

19. "Hepatitis B Disease and Vaccine Facts." National Vaccine Information Center, Available online http://www.nvic.org/ Diseases/hepBfacts.htm

20. "Hepatitis B Vaccine Reaction Reports Outnumbered Reported Disease Cases in Children According to Vaccine Safety Group." Vaccination News. (January 27, 1999) Available online at http:// www.vaccinationnews.com/scandals/Aug_16_02/Scandal19.htm

21. "Hepatitis B Vaccine victims in France Sue; Schools Suspend Vaccination Program." National Vaccination Information Center. Available online at http://nvic.org/Diseases/hepbfrance.htm

22. "VAERS Reports on Deaths – For Hep B vaccine" Testimonies of the report are available online at http://www.whale.to/v/vaers_ reports.html

23. Classen, J.B.: Diabetes epidemic follows hepatitis B immunization program. *New Zealand Medical Journal*, 109: 195, 1996

24. Todar, K. "Haemophilus influenzae" (2004) University of Wisconsin-Madison Department of Bacteriology. Article online at http://www.textbookofbacteriology.net/haemophilus.html

25. "Haemophilus Influenzae type b" Health Professionals, Online Resource Center. New Zealand Immunization Advisor Center. Available online at http://www.immune.org.nz/?t=640

26. "Child Health USA – 2000-2006 – Vaccine Preventable Diseases." U.S Department of Health and Human Services. Maternal and Child Health Bureau. Available online at http://mchb.hrsa.gov/ chusa02/main_pages/page_02.htm

27. Berkovitch, M., Bulkowstein, M., Zhovtis, D., Greenberg, R., Nitzan, Y., Barzilay, B., Boldur, I. "Colonization rate of bacteria in the throat of healthy infants." *International Journal*

of Pediatric Otorhinolaryngology, Volume 63, Number 1, 15 March 2002 , pp. 19-24(6)

28. "Vaccine Information: Measels, Mumps and Rubella" National Network for Immunization Information. (2006) Available online http://www.immunizationinfo.org/vaccineInfo/vaccine_detail. cfv?id=24

29. "Recommended Immunization Schedule for Persons Aged 0-6 Years – United States – 2008" Center for Disease Control and Prevention. Effective December 1, 2007 Available online http:// www.cispimmunize.org/IZSchedule_Childhood.pdf

30. "Child Health USA – 2006. Incidence of Select Vaccine-Preventable Diseases Among Children Under Age 5: 2004." Source: Centers for Disease Control and Prevention. Summary of notifiable diseases: United States, 2004. MMWR, Vol. 53, No. 53; 2006. Online at http://mchb.hrsa.gov/chusa_06/healthstat/ children/graphs/0311vpd.htm

31. "Rubella, Measles, Mumps." Health Professionals Online Resource Center. Immunization Advisory Center. New Zealand. (Source: Immunization Handbook 2006) Available online http:// www.immune.org.nz/?t=642

32. "Vaccine-Preventable Childhood Diseases." Centers for Disease Control and Prevention. Online at http://www.cdc.gov/vaccines/ vpd-vac/child-vpd.htm

33. Berkovitch, M., Bulkowstein, M., Zhovtis, D., Greenberg, R., Nitzan, Y., Barzilay, B., Boldur, I. "Colonization rate of bacteria in the throat of healthy infants." *International Journal of Pediatric Otorhinolaryngology*, Volume 63, Number 1, 15 March 2002 , pp. 19-24(6)

34. Feikin, D., Schuchat, A., et.al.. "Mortality from invasive pneumococcal pneumonia in the era of antibiotic resistance, 1995-1997." *American Journal of Public Health.* V90.(2); Feb 2000

35. Eskola, J. et al., "Efficacy of a pneumococcal conjugate vaccine against acute otitis media," *New England Journal of Medicine*, 344:403-409, February 8, 2001. [PubMed Abstract]

36. Miller, JD. "The Replacement Effect: Concern over a vaccine

that causes unintended increase in related infections." Pediatric Infectious Disease Unit at Soroka University Medical Center in Beer-Sheva, Israel

37. Miller, J.D. "Unblocking the vaccine pipeline," *The Scientist*, May 13, 2003. http://www.biomedcentral.com/news/20030513/02/

38. Strickler, H, Rosenberg, P, Devesa, S, Hertel, J, Fraumeni, J, Goedert, J (1998). "Contamination of poliovirus vaccines with simian virus 40 (1955-1963) and subsequent cancer rates." *JAMA* 279 (4): 292-5.

39. Kops, SP. "Oral polio vaccine and human cancer: a reassessment of SV40 as a contaminant based upon legal documents." *Anticancer Research*. 2000 Nov-Dec; 20(6C):4745-9.

40. The Advisory Committee on Immunization Practices. Notice to readers: recommended childhood immunization schedule – United States, 2000. *MMWR Weekly* January 21, 2000; 49(02):35-38, 47.

41. World Health Organization. 2003. "Introduction of inactivated poliovirus vaccine into oral poliovirus vaccine-using countries." W.H.O. position paper. Wkly. *Epidemiol. Rec.* 78:241-250.

42. "International Notes Certification of Poliomyelitis Eradication - the Americas, 1994." Morbidity and Mortality Weekly Report (1994) 43 (39): 720–2. Centers for Disease Control and Prevention. PMID 7522302.

43. "Europe achieves historic milestone as Region is declared polio-free." European Region of the World Health Organization (2002-06-21). Press release. http://www.who.int/mediacentre/news/releases/releaseeuro02/en/index.html

44. "Lightening Safety - Updated AMS Recommendations for Lightning Safety - 2002" National Weather Service. Available online at http://www.lightningsafety.noaa.gov/ams_lightning_rec.htm

45. "Travelers' Health: Yellow Book. Chapter 4: Prevention on Specific Infectious Diseases, Poliomyelitis." CDC Health Information for International Travel 2008. Online at http://wwwn.cdc.gov/travel/yellowBookCh4-Poliomyelitis.aspx

46. Cullen, R. M., Walker, W.J. "Poliovirus in New Zealand 1915-

1997" Original Research Paper. June 1999, Online at http://www. rnzcgp.org.nz/news/nzfp/June1999/orrc.htm

47. "Poliomyelitis" World Health Organization. Polio Fact Sheets. January 2008, Available online at http://www.who.int/ mediacentre/factsheets/fs114/en/

Index

About the Author

Murray C. Clarke, ND., D.Hom., M.Hom., L.Ac.

Dr. Murray Clarke is originally from New Zealand and moved to America in 1984 to study medicine. He now holds licenses and doctorates in three fields of medicine: naturopathic medicine, homeopathic medicine and Chinese medicine (including acupuncture and herbology).

Dr. Clarke's clinic is located in Santa Monica, California, where for the past 20 years he has helped to pioneer the field of holistic pediatrics, earning recognition as a leading holistic specialist for children in the Los Angeles area.

The private medical clinic opened in 1988 with a general practice utilizing acupuncture, herbs, nutrition and homeopathy. Mothers and fathers who experienced restored and robust good health after treatment began bringing their infants and children to be treated. With the same measure of benefits and success working with children, Dr. Clarke's reputation continued to grow within the community, and local M.D. pediatricians began referring their own patients to him when they were unable to help with standard pharmaceutical approaches.

Dr. Clarke has continued to focus his experience, treatments and quest for knowledge on what causes ill-health in children and how to treat and cure the roots of these maladies in the safest and most effective manner. Due to this dedication, Dr. Clarke has earned the success and reputation of being the most sought and well-known homeopathic pediatrician in Los Angeles.

In 2000, Dr. Murray Clarke founded the company *ChildLife Essentials* ® www.childlife.net , formulating and manufacturing the first complete line of nutritional supplements exclusively for infants and children. These products are now distributed and sold in pharmacies, health food stores and Whole Foods stores throughout America, as well as internationally distributed in Europe, Asia and the South Pacific.

CPSIA information can be obtained at www.ICGtesting.com
Printed in the USA
BVOW11s1943100414

350253BV00005B/12/P

9 781935 953050